A Mastery Approach to Complex Esophageal Diseases

Dmitry Oleynikov • P. Marco Fisichella
Editors

A Mastery Approach to Complex Esophageal Diseases

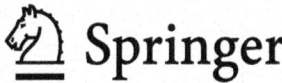 Springer

Editors
Dmitry Oleynikov
Nebraska Medical Center
University of Nebraska Medical Center
Omaha
Nebraska
USA

P. Marco Fisichella
Harvard Medical School
West Roxbury
Massachusetts
USA

ISBN 978-3-030-09328-0   ISBN 978-3-319-75795-7   (eBook)
https://doi.org/10.1007/978-3-319-75795-7

This Springer imprint is published by the registered company Springer International Publishing AG part
of Springer Nature
The registered company address is: Gewerbestrasse 11, 6330 Cham, Switzerland

Contents

Introduction: "A Mastery Approach to Complex Esophageal Diseases"

Over the last few decades, many concepts about esophageal surgery and the diseases that we treat have changed dramatically. Advances in technology and the development of new surgical and diagnostic tools have changed the approach to esophageal diseases. Standardization of disease classification with the adoption of the newly revised Chicago Classification in conjunction with the widespread use of high-resolution manometry has resulted in newer diagnostic criteria for both hypomotility disorders and hypercontractility disorders, leading to the expansion of surgical therapy for achalasia. New endoluminal approaches for esophageal disease, such as POEM (per-oral endoscopic myotomy), have gained greater visibility over the last few years, and although more knowledge and awareness of this procedure exists, its effectiveness compared to standard techniques remains debatable. Robotic-assisted surgeries have also grown in the field of general surgery, and procedures like robotic-assisted Heller Myotomy are increasingly more common. Endoscopic ultrasound and endoluminal, laparoscopic, and thoracoscopic approaches are being utilized much more frequently in the diagnostic approach to benign esophageal tumors. Gastroesophageal reflux disease (GERD) remains an extremely common gastrointestinal disease, requiring a significant portion of health care resources for effective treatment and management. Newer treatment modalities have been introduced for GERD, including a variety of endoluminal devices and therapies. These have allowed for more noninvasive approaches, including endoluminal ablation and endoscopic mucosal resection, resulting in a significant change in the standard treatment of Barrett esophagus. Recently, more focus has centered on the role of anti-reflux surgery after bariatric procedures. Sleeve gastrectomy as the bariatric surgery of choice could be a contributing factor in the rise of de novo postsurgical GERD. This has resulted in an increased need for revisional Roux-en-Y gastric bypass procedures and has renewed interest in the development of new therapies for symptomatic and postsurgical GERD. It is my distinct pleasure to have a very distinguished group of scientists contribute to this innovative issue.

The management of esophageal diseases is complex and continually changing, and each expert has focused on important topics that speak to us all about the ongoing challenges in the treatment of these diseases.

Omaha, NE, USA   Dmitry Oleynikov, M.D.
Boston, MA, USA   P. Marco Fisichella, M.D., M.B.A.

Non-operative Treatment of Gastroesophageal Reflux Disease

1

Adarsh M. Thaker and V. Raman Muthusamy

Physiology and Pathophysiology of GERD

Gastroesophageal reflux occurs when there is loss of the natural anti-reflux barrier at the gastroesophageal junction (GEJ). Some degree of reflux is considered physiologic, but when this process causes troublesome symptoms and/or complications, the condition is defined as gastroesophageal reflux disease (GERD) [1].

The fundamental mechanisms producing reflux are transient lower esophageal sphincter relaxations (TLESRs) and decreased lower esophageal sphincter (LES) pressure, which have been shown to occur physiologically in asymptomatic subjects [2]. A third factor is anatomic disruption of the GEJ, the natural antireflux barrier, which may occur due to the presence of a hiatal hernia, scleroderma, or after myotomy for the treatment of achalasia. Esophageal dysmotility, which can be severe in 20–30% of patients, is associated with more severe reflux, worse mucosal injury, and severe respiratory symptoms due to decreased clearance of refluxed contents [3, 4]. Gastroparesis has also been linked to GERD, potentially due to direct reflux of poorly cleared gastric contents into the esophagus or by distension of the proximal stomach triggering TLESRs [5].

These disturbances allow abnormal acid exposure on the esophageal mucosa, particularly in times of increased acid secretion after meals. Despite some buffering of gastric acid by ingested food, the acid forms a layer on top of the food in the proximal stomach, forming a so-called "acid pocket" which refluxes into the distal esophagus. This reservoir appears to primarily contribute to GERD in most patients rather than acid hypersecretion [4].

A. M. Thaker, M.D. (✉) · V. R. Muthusamy, M.D., F.A.C.G., F.A.S.G.E.
Vatche and Tamar Manoukian Division of Digestive Diseases,
David Geffen School of Medicine at UCLA, Los Angeles, CA, USA
e-mail: athaker@mednet.ucla.edu; raman@mednet.ucla.edu

© Springer International Publishing AG, part of Springer Nature 2018
D. Oleynikov, P. M. Fisichella (eds.), *A Mastery Approach to Complex Esophageal Diseases*, https://doi.org/10.1007/978-3-319-75795-7_1

Multiple factors have been shown to decrease LES tone and/or increase the number of TLESRs on physiologic testing. Dietary agents include fatty foods, chocolate, coffee, tobacco, alcohol, and carminatives (such as peppermint and other agents with essential oils) [6, 7]. Other factors associated with increased esophageal acid exposure and symptomatic reflux include sleep, belching, pregnancy, exogenous estrogen, certain medications (i.e. calcium channel blockers, nitrates, muscle relaxants), and exercise [8–12]. Obesity in particular appears to exaggerate all of the proposed pathophysiologic mechanisms [4].

Clinical Presentation of GERD

In order to streamline clinical practice and investigations regarding GERD, it has been divided into several clinical syndromes by the Montreal definition and classification by consensus (Fig. 1.1). The two major subgroups are esophageal and extraesophageal syndromes. The esophageal syndromes include (1) symptomatic syndromes (subdivided into typical reflux symptoms and chest pain syndrome), and (2) syndromes with esophageal injury (esophagitis, stricture, Barrett's Esophagus [BE], and esophageal adenocarcinoma). The extraesophageal syndromes are subdivided by the level of evidence supporting their association with atypical manifestations.

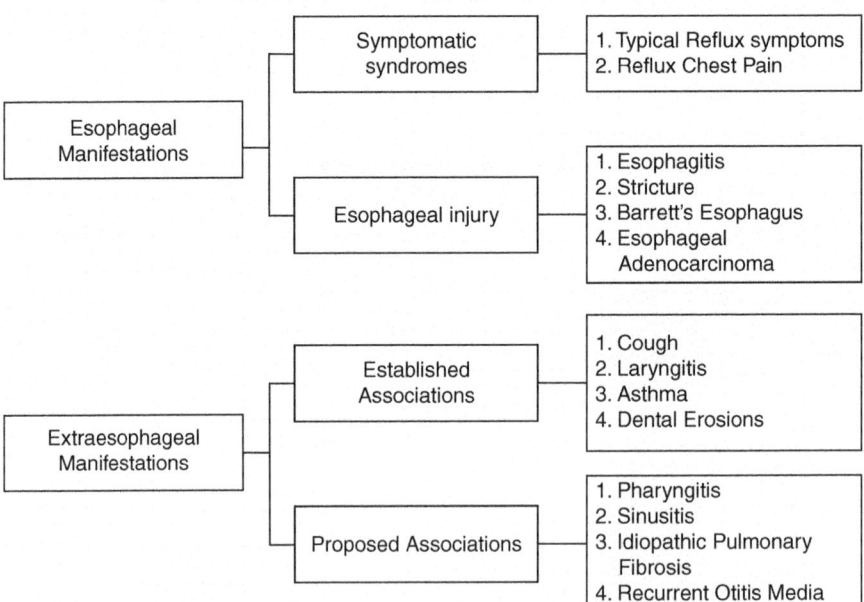

Fig. 1.1 The Montreal Classification of the constituent syndromes of GERD. GERD is defined as a condition which develops when the reflux of gastric contents causes troublesome symptoms or complications [1]

The characteristic symptoms of typical GERD are retrosternal burning, commonly known as "heartburn," and regurgitation, defined as the perception of flow of gastric contents into the mouth or hypopharynx [1]. Other symptoms attributed to GERD include angina-like chest pain, dysphagia (especially in the presence of severe esophagitis or stricture), and water brash (the sudden appearance of a salty or sour fluid in the mouth from the salivary glands in response to intraesophageal acid exposure) [1, 13]. Atypical or extraesophageal manifestations of GERD may include cough, asthma, chronic laryngitis (also called laryngopharyngeal reflux or LPR), hoarseness, and sinusitis. However, these are felt to be multifactorial disease processes in which reflux can be an aggravating factor, rather than the sole cause [1]. Practical, cost-effective methods to identify the subgroup of patients for whom GERD truly plays a causal role in these conditions or to determine which patients may respond to acid-suppressive therapy are still required [14–17].

Complications of GERD

Erosive esophagitis, defined as esophageal mucosal ulceration or erosion on endoscopy, is among the most predominant complications of GERD with a reported prevalence ranging from 6% to 30% [18]. Patients may present with retrosternal pain, dysphagia, or anemia from chronic blood loss. It appears to be caused by a combination of reflux of gastric contents, poor esophageal clearance of the refluxed material, and impairment of resistance mechanisms which protect against mucosal damage [19]. Esophagitis can occur transiently and/or in asymptomatic patients, and is rated as severe in 20% of cases [5, 18].

A consequence of esophagitis is the development of peptic strictures due to the deposition of collagen and scar formation, which can contract over time and narrow the esophageal lumen. Clinically, peptic strictures can remain asymptomatic or present as dysphagia or food bolus impaction. They may require endoscopic dilation followed by long-term maintenance acid-suppression to prevent recurrence [20, 21].

GERD is also an established risk factor for esophageal adenocarcinoma and its precursor, BE, characterized by changes in the esophageal squamous mucosa to a specialized columnar epithelium, intestinal metaplasia [22]. The prevailing belief is that malignancy develops through a series of consecutive changes promoted by GERD, from erosive esophagitis to non-dysplastic BE, low-grade dysplasia, high-grade dysplasia, adenocarcinoma in situ, and invasive esophageal adenocarcinoma [22].

Diagnostic Procedures

Proton-Pump Inhibitor (PPI) Trial

GERD is diagnosed presumptively on the basis of typical symptoms of heartburn or regurgitation, and initiation of empiric treatment with a proton pump inhibitor (PPI) in this setting is recommended [23]. A meta-analysis demonstrated that a response to empiric PPI therapy had a sensitivity of 78% and specificity of 54% [24]. However, the sensitivity of these symptoms for the presence of erosive esophagitis ranges between 30% and 76% and the specificity ranges from 62% to 96% [23, 25]. Therefore, a PPI trial is a reasonable initial step for patients presenting with typical symptoms without alarm features but does not necessarily exclude complicated disease or alternative diagnoses.

Upper Endoscopy

Universal endoscopy for patients with GERD is not recommended or cost effective, as the vast majority of patients will have normal endoscopic findings [13, 23, 26, 27]. Less than 65% of the minority of patients who do undergo upper endoscopy were shown to have abnormal findings [18, 23]. Relative to the prevalence of GERD in the population, the prevalence of clinically significant findings which would alter the clinical course or management of these patients is low.

The indications for upper endoscopy in GERD (Table 1.1) are under continued debate, with slightly varying recommendations from society guidelines [23, 26–28]. Endoscopy is generally recommended on initial presentation for patients presenting with alarm features suggestive of complicated disease, such as stricture, esophagitis, or malignancy. The alarm features include dysphagia, odynophagia, bleeding, involuntary weight loss, epigastric mass, recurrent vomiting, or anemia [23, 26–29].

Endoscopy is also indicated for patients with persistent or progressive GERD symptoms despite appropriate medical therapy (i.e. 4–8 weeks of twice-daily empiric PPI therapy taken appropriately) [26, 27]. Routine esophageal biopsies are not recommended specifically to diagnose GERD but are recommended to evaluate for complications of GERD, such as suspected BE, dysplasia, or malignancy [23]. Biopsies are also suggested to evaluate for eosinophilic esophagitis (EoE) in patients presenting with dysphagia, even with a normal endoscopy, although a subset of such patients may have an overlap with GERD and respond to PPI treatment, thereby termed, PPI-responsive EoE (PPI-REE) [23, 28].

Table 1.1 Indications for endoscopy in patients with GERD [23, 26]

Non-response twice daily PPI trial for 4–8 weeks
Dysphagia or odynophagia
Involuntary weight loss
Evidence of GI bleeding or anemia
Palpable mass on physical exam or finding of mass, ulcer, or stricture on imaging study
Persistent vomiting (7–10 days)
Screening for Barrett's esophagus in selected patients, if clinically indicated, including as follow-up of treated erosive esophagitis
Evaluation before or for recurrent symptoms after antireflux procedures
Placement of wireless pH monitoring

Upper endoscopy is indicated as a screening test for BE in men with chronic GERD (>5 years) and/or at least weekly symptoms with two or more risk factors for BE or esophageal adenocarcinoma including: Age >50 years, Caucasian race, central obesity, current or past history of smoking, and a confirmed family history of BE or esophageal adenocarcinoma in a first-degree relative [30]. Endoscopy is also indicated in patients who have erosive esophagitis on a prior endoscopy after a period of twice daily PPI therapy since BE can be identified in as many as 12% of these patients after healing [26, 31]. Finally, endoscopy is often performed for preoperative evaluation in patients being considered for anti-reflux surgery or for wireless esophageal pH monitoring [26].

There is little data to support endoscopy in the evaluation for GERD without alarm features, for extra-esophageal manifestations, or for BE screening in women due to the low prevalence of significant findings [26].

pH and Impedance Testing

In addition to upper endoscopy, patients who fail twice daily PPI dosing should undergo esophageal pH testing in order to verify the diagnosis and to assess for possible causes for refractory symptoms. This can be performed via ambulatory intranasal catheter (with or without impedance testing) or wireless pH probe monitoring with a portable data recorder for patients to record symptom events. This allows for providers to establish symptom-reflux association through validated parameters such as the Symptom Index and the Symptom Association Probability [32].

Multichannel intraluminal impedance (MII), which when combined with pH testing (MII-pH), enables detection of gastroesophageal reflux of both acid and non-acid contents [32, 33]. Impedance measures resistance to electrical current flow between metallic rings mounted on a catheter and decreases in the presence of refluxed gastric liquid, which has good electrical conductance. Measurement of impedance at multiple sites (i.e. using a multichannel catheter) over time allows for the establishment of bolus flow directionality, including the proximal reflux of gastric contents into the esophagus [32, 33]. Coupled with pH measurements, impedance testing helps clarify (1) whether the recorded pH change represents retrograde bolus (reflux) or anterograde bolus (ingested food), (2) whether reflux events are associated with symptom events, and (3) whether the refluxed contents represent acid or non-acid (alkaline) reflux [32].

Whether to perform pH testing on or off PPI therapy is an important initial decision in planning the study. It depends on the clinical presentation and the question to be answered. Except in specific circumstances, pH testing should be performed off therapy (with PPI discontinued for at least 7 days preceding the study) since most validation studies on pH monitoring were performed under this condition [32]. Impedance-pH testing on medications also does not reliably confirm the presence of GERD in patients referred for antireflux surgery, so it is recommended these patients undergo testing off treatment [34].

Testing off PPI is primarily used to verify the diagnosis of GERD since it reflects the natural esophageal acid exposure without interference from treatment. This also results in more symptoms and therefore a higher yield of symptom-reflux associations [32]. Testing on PPI is indicated for patients with obvious evidence of acid reflux, such as severe esophagitis, peptic stricture, BE, or prior positive pH testing, to evaluate for ongoing acid or non-acid reflux to assess for treatment failure [32]. A third alternative is the 96 h wireless pH study, beginning with 48 h off treatment to verify the diagnosis of GERD followed by 48 h on treatment to evaluate whether breakthrough acid exposure despite PPI explains their symptoms [35].

Mucosal Impedance

Mucosal impedance (MI) is a promising new technology to aid in the diagnosis of GERD and assessment of treatment response. The MI catheter is applied to the esophageal mucosa during endoscopy for immediate and rapid measurement. MI is related to the presence of dilated intercellular spaces (DIS), a histologic feature of GERD which affects para-cellular permeability. Increased permeability results in decreased MI [33]. Preliminary testing has shown that MI can differentiate GERD (with or without esophagitis) from EoE and non-GERD related conditions (including normal esophagus and achalasia). MI has been shown to have a superior specificity for GERD compared to pH monitoring (95% vs. 64%) as well as a superior positive predictive value (96% vs. 40%) with a similar sensitivity and negative predictive value [33, 36].

MI technology obtains information more rapidly than ambulatory pH testing and may serve as a better reflection of chronic disease in its correlation with histologic changes rather than isolated events. Impedance values recover to normal in patients with GERD after PPI therapy, suggesting MI can be used to monitor acid suppression and treatment response. It may also be useful to predict likely responders to anti-reflux procedures. Finally, it may help clarify whether a patient's extraesophageal symptoms are truly reflux related [33]. Larger validation studies and wider availability of this nascent technology are eagerly awaited.

Radiographs

Imaging with barium esophagram can be helpful in patients with dysphagia to evaluate for stricture, but due to its poor sensitivity for reflux or esophagitis, it is not recommended as a diagnostic test in GERD [30].

Management of GERD

Lifestyle Modifications

Lifestyle modifications suggested for GERD include dietary and behavioral changes. Avoidance of foods and substances that can cause reflux episodes or (e.g. chocolate, coffee, tobacco, alcohol, peppermint, carbonated beverages) or those that can produce symptoms (e.g. citrus and tomato products, spicy foods) is often suggested [37]. Behavioral modifications include weight loss, smoking cessation, avoiding large meals, avoiding recumbence right after meals, and head of bed elevation [37]. However, the data supporting each of these practices is mixed, especially for patients with frequent or severe symptoms. On systematic review, the strongest evidence supports weight loss and head of bed elevation, although smoking cessation is recommended for its global health benefits as well [37]. Universal application of these lifestyle measures are not practical, particularly without a sacrifice in quality of life. It is therefore recommended that specific lifestyle modifications are tailored to individual patients instead of global implementation (e.g. weight loss for overweight or obese patients; head of bed elevation for patients with symptoms when recumbent; or identification and avoidance of specific trigger foods rather than a full elimination diet) [28, 37].

Antacids, Mucosal Protectants, and Prokinetic Agents

Antacids such as sodium bicarbonate, magnesium hydroxide, aluminum hydroxide, and calcium carbonate can provide symptom relief by neutralizing intragastric acid. They have the most rapid onset of action of GERD treatments. However, due to their short duration of action and the risks of excess use (e.g. milk-alkali syndrome from calcium carbonate), direct antacids are generally reserved for on-demand treatment in patients with mild and infrequent symptoms [28].

Sucralfate (sucrose-aluminum sulfate) is a mucosal protectant believed to reduce symptoms by decreasing esophageal acid exposure. Sucralfate's short duration of action and lower efficacy compared to anti-secretory agents limits its use. It appears to be useful as a first line agent with or without antacids for mild intermittent symptoms in women who are pregnant or lactating [38]. There does not appear to be a role for sucralfate in the non-pregnant GERD patient [23].

Alginate (sodium alginate) is a seaweed based agent which forms a gel raft in the proximal stomach on top of an ingested meal, co-localizing with the acid pocket. This creates a barrier that prevents the acid from reaching the esophagus and thereby reduces acid-related injury and symptoms [39]. Alginate appears to be less effective than PPIs and H2RAs, but more effective than antacids [40]. It also appears to be more effective as combination therapy with H2RAs compared to H2RAs alone which makes it potentially useful to patients who are intolerant or averse to PPIs but ineffectively treated with H2RAs alone [39].

Prokinetics such as metoclopramide are associated with increased adverse events and do not have a role in the management of GERD except transiently if there is concomitant gastroparesis. Metoclopramide has a black box warning for tardive dyskinesia and treatment greater than 12 weeks should be avoided. Another agent not commercially available in the United States is domperidone, which is associated with QT prolongation and cardiac arrhythmias [23].

Histamine 2 Receptor Antagonists

Histamine 2 receptor antagonists (H2RAs) or "H2-blockers" (i.e. cimetidine, ranitidine, famotidine) reduce acid secretion from parietal cells by inhibiting activation by histamine, which is released in a paracrine fashion by nearby enterochromaffin-like cells [41]. The principle limitation of H2RAs as maintenance therapy for GERD is the development of tolerance (tachyphylaxis) as early as 1–2 weeks of therapy in some patients [42–44]. H2RAs also have limited efficacy in healing erosive esophagitis compared with PPIs [45]. Therefore, they are generally suggested for short-duration or as-needed treatment for patients with mild, intermittent symptoms and no esophageal complications. H2RAs can also be considered as maintenance therapy for the subset of patients without erosive disease who experience heartburn relief without tachyphylaxis [23].

H2RAs are commonly added at bedtime to patients with persistent or nocturnal symptoms despite twice daily PPI dosing. This has been shown physiologically to further improve nocturnal gastric acid levels or breakthrough in patients already twice-daily PPI doses [42, 46]. However, this practice has been called into question because improved nocturnal gastric acid levels do not necessarily result in decreased esophageal acid exposure and these studies did not address the development of tolerance to H2RAs [47]. Acid suppression with the addition of nocturnal H2RAs was found to decrease significantly after only 1 week of therapy and fell to pre-H2RA levels after 1 month of therapy due to tolerance [44]. However, for unexplained reasons, some patients maintained some degree of improved acid control chronically [44, 47]. Therefore, a small subset of patients may potentially benefit from nocturnal H2RA in combination with twice daily PPI but it is not recommended as a standard approach. Furthermore, patients who do not respond to twice daily PPI should be considered for additional diagnostic evaluations rather than relying on H2RA addition as an extended therapeutic trial.

Proton Pump Inhibitors

Proton pump inhibitors (PPIs) inhibit gastric acid secretion by selectively inactivating the H+/K+ ATPase "proton pump" on parietal cells. PPIs are prodrugs which require acid activation, absorption into the bloodstream, and active proton pumps in order to bind to them and exert their effects. They covalently bind to active proton pumps for a longer duration of effect, but their bloodstream half-life is relatively short (~90–120 min). PPIs therefore achieve maximum efficacy when the peak bloodstream concentration coincides with activation of proton pumps during a meal (especially a protein meal). For this reason, most PPIs are ideally taken before meals. On one hand, acid suppression by PPIs is increased in the setting of a meal when compared to the fasting state [48]. On the other hand, the absorption and bioavailability of PPIs are diminished when they are administered at the same time as a meal [49]. PPIs are therefore recommended to be taken in a relatively narrow window of time, ideally 30–60 min prior to a meal, in order to achieve maximum acid suppression [23].

A newer PPI dexlansoprazole provides an exception to the need for meal timing adherence. It has a dual-delayed release formulation using two sets of enteric coated capsules designed to maintain bloodstream concentrations for longer periods of time [49]. This medication can therefore be given irrespective of meals or the timing of meals. Another agent known as VECAM is a combination of omeprazole and succinic acid, which was shown to induce gastric acid secretion. The addition of succinic acid thereby eliminates the need for a subsequent meal after taking the PPI and appeared to be more effective than omeprazole alone in a preclinical study [50].

PPIs are highly effective in the management of GERD and its complications. PPIs are associated with superior healing rates and decreased relapse rates for erosive esophagitis compared to H2RAs (84% vs. 52%) [23, 51]. For non-erosive reflux disease, PPIs have demonstrated superiority over H2RAs for heartburn relief with a relative risk for heartburn remission of 0.66 (95% confidence interval [CI] 0.60–0.73) on direct comparison [52].

In a review of clinical studies, the relative potencies of PPIs based on mean 24 h gastric pH compared to omeprazole were 0.23, 0.90, 1.0, 1.60, and 1.82 for pantoprazole, lansoprazole, omeprazole, esomeprazole, and rabeprazole, respectively [53]. Despite the differences in potency and statistical evidence of superiority of some agents over others, symptom relief among the PPIs appears to be similar and the clinical significance of other differences is minimal [54]. There is limited but inconsistent evidence to support the use of one PPI over another for erosive esophagitis, but the relative potencies can be taken into consideration for PPI selection for patients with refractory symptoms or inflammation [4, 55, 56].

Initial PPI therapy for most patients with typical reflux should start with once daily dosing, taken before the first meal of the day. For patients with partial symptom relief or predominately nocturnal symptoms, options include moving the dose to before dinner, twice daily dosing before the first and last meals of the day, or a one-time trial of an alternative PPI [23]. Since approximately 70% of proton pumps are activated during each meal for PPIs to bind, patients should be advised that it may take up to 5 days to reach steady state effect and to assess symptom relief [57]. For patients with good symptom response for 8–12 weeks, a trial off medications can be considered. Patients may develop rebound acid hypersecretion with abrupt discontinuation of PPIs, so a taper is generally recommended [41]. Patients with recurrent symptoms during the taper can be stepped up one degree to the minimum effective dose required for relief.

Adverse Events of PPI

The most commonly reported side effects of PPIs are headache, diarrhea, and abdominal discomfort. These can usually be mitigated by dose reduction or switching to another PPI [23, 28]. PPIs are considered safe in pregnancy if clinically indicated [23, 38].

There has been significant attention given recently to the association between PPIs and a variety of other conditions, including kidney disease, dementia, osteoporosis, myocardial infarction, small intestinal bacterial overgrowth, spontaneous bacterial peritonitis, *Clostridium difficile* infection, pneumonia, micronutrient deficiencies, and gastrointestinal malignancies [58, 59]. The evidence to support these observations largely emerges from low or very low quality, mostly observational studies, and higher quality data has often refuted the observed differences [58, 59]. Furthermore, the absolute risk of many of these conditions remains low despite seemingly high relative risk estimates [58].

However, these studies have highlighted the important fact that PPIs are frequently overused for inappropriate conditions. This has resulted in increased healthcare costs and exposure to potential adverse events. When used for appropriate conditions and for the correct duration, the benefits of PPI therapy far outweigh the risks and there is no definite evidence to support a change in management [4, 58, 59]. However, modest increases in risk become more important in the setting of inappropriate PPI use because there is no benefit [58].

In general, long-term PPI use is appropriate in the setting of symptomatic typical GERD or the presence of the complications of GERD, such as esophagitis, peptic strictures, or BE. Long-term PPI therapy is appropriate in patients with PPI-responsive symptoms, although a taper to the lowest effective dose, on demand dosing, or intermittent dosing (i.e. 2–4 weeks at a time) should be considered [4, 59]. A subset of patients may also successfully be tapered to daily H2RA if they do not experience tachyphylaxis [23].

Potassium-Competitive Acid Blockers

Potassium-competitive acid blockers (P-CABs) are a class of acid-suppressive medications which, like PPIs, inhibit the gastric H+/K+-ATPase proton pump but do so in a potassium competitive, reversible manner. The advantages of P-CABs are that their binding is unaffected by the acid secretion state, and therefore dosing can be meal independent. These agents include revaprazan and vonoprazan and are not currently available outside of Asia. Initial investigations on vonoprazan reported a more rapid, potent, and prolonged inhibition of acid secretion compared to PPIs [60, 61]. Additional clinical studies are underway.

Refractory GERD

The reported rates of patients reporting persistent troublesome heartburn or regurgitation despite PPI therapy have ranged as high as 40–50% [62, 63]. Several survey studies have also shown that compliance to recommended therapy is poor [23, 63, 64]. Furthermore, adherence to recommended timing—at least 15 min and ideally 30–60 min before a meal—is also poor, and over half of all patients may be suboptimally dosing their treatment [63]. Providers may be partly to blame, as an earlier survey of physicians revealed high rates of incorrect dosing instructions [23]. Therefore, an initial step in the management of patients with potentially refractory GERD should be assessment of compliance, adherence to medication timing, and optimization of therapy.

Patients with refractory symptoms despite PPI therapy should undergo upper endoscopy to evaluate for esophageal complications or alternative diagnoses to explain their symptoms. This includes biopsy for EoE, even in the setting of normal endoscopy [23]. They should also undergo pH or pH-impedance monitoring, which can help identify a diagnosis alternative to non-erosive reflux disease but with overlapping symptoms.

Assuming a normal endoscopy and exclusion of EoE and motility disorders, potential diagnoses include esophageal hypersensitivity and functional heartburn. Patients with a positive correlation between reflux events and but whose acid exposure parameters remain within normal limits are considered to have esophageal hypersensitivity. Patients no correlation of symptoms with reflux events are considered to have functional heartburn [18]. For unclear reasons, as many as 50% of patients with functional heartburn respond to PPI therapy, perhaps due to misclassification [18]. Additional therapies for functional heartburn include lifestyle modifications through identification of triggers and psychosocial associations, neuromodulation through agents such as tricyclic antidepressants or selective serotonin reuptake inhibitors (SSRIs), or alternative therapies such as acupuncture [18].

Medical treatment options for patients with refractory GERD verified by pH testing are limited, particularly because PPIs are highly effective in most patients. Increasing the PPI from once daily to twice daily dosing or a single trial of an alternative, more potent agent can be considered. Addition of bedtime H2RA in a therapeutic trial to identify the subset of patients who may not become tolerant can also be attempted. Agents such as baclofen, metoclopramide, and domperidone have been suggested but are limited by side effects and/or availability [23]. Truly PPI refractory patients may therefore be good candidates for antireflux procedures.

References

1. Vakil N, van Zanten SV, Kahrilas P, Dent J, Jones R, Global Consensus G. The Montreal definition and classification of gastroesophageal reflux disease: a global evidence-based consensus. Am J Gastroenterol. 2006;101(8):1900–20; quiz 43. https://doi.org/10.1111/j.1572-0241.2006.00630.x.
2. Wallin L, Madsen T. 12-hour simultaneous registration of acid reflex and peristaltic activity in the oesophagus. A study in normal subjects. Scand J Gastroenterol. 1979;14(5):561–6.
3. Diener U, Patti MG, Molena D, Fisichella PM, Way LW. Esophageal dysmotility and gastroesophageal reflux disease. J Gastrointest Surg. 2001;5(3):260–5.
4. Scarpignato C, Gatta L, Zullo A, Blandizzi C, Group S-A-F, Italian Society of Pharmacology tIAoHG, et al. Effective and safe proton pump inhibitor therapy in acid-related diseases - a position paper addressing benefits and potential harms of acid suppression. BMC Med. 2016;14(1):179. https://doi.org/10.1186/s12916-016-0718-z.

5. Richter JE, Rubenstein JH. Presentation and epidemiology of gastroesophageal reflux disease. Gastroenterology. 2017. doi:https://doi.org/10.1053/j.gastro.2017.07.045.
6. Vitale GC, Cheadle WG, Patel B, Sadek SA, Michel ME, Cuschieri A. The effect of alcohol on nocturnal gastroesophageal reflux. JAMA. 1987;258(15):2077–9.
7. Nebel OT, Castell DO. Lower esophageal sphincter pressure changes after food ingestion. Gastroenterology. 1972;63(5):778–83.
8. Derakhshan MH, Robertson EV, Fletcher J, Jones GR, Lee YY, Wirz AA, et al. Mechanism of association between BMI and dysfunction of the gastro-oesophageal barrier in patients with normal endoscopy. Gut. 2012;61(3):337–43. https://doi.org/10.1136/gutjnl-2011-300633.
9. Barham CP, Gotley DC, Mills A, Alderson D. Precipitating causes of acid reflux episodes in ambulant patients with gastro-oesophageal reflux disease. Gut. 1995;36(4):505–10.
10. Herregods TV, van Hoeij FB, Oors JM, Bredenoord AJ, Smout AJ. Effect of running on gastroesophageal reflux and reflux mechanisms. Am J Gastroenterol. 2016;111(7):940–6. https://doi.org/10.1038/ajg.2016.122.
11. Gerson LB, Fass R. A systematic review of the definitions, prevalence, and response to treatment of nocturnal gastroesophageal reflux disease. Clin Gastroenterol Hepatol. 2009;7(4):372–8; quiz 67. https://doi.org/10.1016/j.cgh.2008.11.021.
12. Zheng Z, Margolis KL, Liu S, Tinker LF, Ye W. Effects of estrogen with and without progestin and obesity on symptomatic gastroesophageal reflux. Gastroenterology. 2008;135(1):72–81. https://doi.org/10.1053/j.gastro.2008.03.039.
13. Richter JE. Typical and atypical presentations of gastroesophageal reflux disease. The role of esophageal testing in diagnosis and management. Gastroenterol Clin N Am. 1996;25(1):75–102.
14. Madanick RD. Extraesophageal presentations of GERD: where is the science? Gastroenterol Clin N Am. 2014;43(1):105–20. https://doi.org/10.1016/j.gtc.2013.11.007.
15. Moore JM, Vaezi MF. Extraesophageal manifestations of gastroesophageal reflux disease: real or imagined? Curr Opin Gastroenterol. 2010;26(4):389–94. https://doi.org/10.1097/MOG.0b013e32833adc8d.
16. Schneider GT, Vaezi MF, Francis DO. Reflux and voice disorders: have we established causality? Curr Otorhinolaryngol Rep. 2016;4(3):157–67. https://doi.org/10.1007/s40136-016-0121-5.
17. Francis DO, Slaughter JC, Ates F, Higginbotham T, Stevens KL, Garrett CG, et al. Airway hypersensitivity, reflux, and phonation contribute to chronic cough. Clin Gastroenterol Hepatol. 2016;14(3):378–84. https://doi.org/10.1016/j.cgh.2015.10.009.
18. Hachem C, Shaheen NJ. Diagnosis and management of functional heartburn. Am J Gastroenterol. 2016;111(1):53–61; quiz 2. https://doi.org/10.1038/ajg.2015.376.
19. Wang R-H. From reflux esophagitis to Barrett's esophagus and esophageal adenocarcinoma. World J Gastroenterol. 2015;21(17):5210–9. https://doi.org/10.3748/wjg.v21.i17.5210.
20. Siddiqui UD, Banerjee S, Barth B, Chauhan SS, Gottlieb KT, Konda V, et al. Tools for endoscopic stricture dilation. Gastrointest Endosc. 2013;78(3):391–404. https://doi.org/10.1016/j.gie.2013.04.170.
21. Siersema PD, de Wijkerslooth LR. Dilation of refractory benign esophageal strictures. Gastrointest Endosc. 2009;70(5):1000–12. https://doi.org/10.1016/j.gie.2009.07.004.
22. Coleman HG, Xie SH, Lagergren J. The epidemiology of esophageal adenocarcinoma. Gastroenterology. 2017. doi:https://doi.org/10.1053/j.gastro.2017.07.046.
23. Katz PO, Gerson LB, Vela MF. Guidelines for the diagnosis and management of gastroesophageal reflux disease. Am J Gastroenterol. 2013;108(3):308–28; quiz 29. https://doi.org/10.1038/ajg.2012.444.
24. Numans ME, Lau J, de Wit NJ, Bonis PA. Short-term treatment with proton-pump inhibitors as a test for gastroesophageal reflux disease: a meta-analysis of diagnostic test characteristics. Ann Intern Med. 2004;140(7):518–27.
25. Moayyedi P, Talley NJ, Fennerty MB, Vakil N. Can the clinical history distinguish between organic and functional dyspepsia? JAMA. 2006;295(13):1566–76. https://doi.org/10.1001/jama.295.13.1566.

26. ASoP C, Muthusamy VR, Lightdale JR, Acosta RD, Chandrasekhara V, Chathadi KV, et al. The role of endoscopy in the management of GERD. Gastrointest Endosc. 2015;81(6):1305–10. https://doi.org/10.1016/j.gie.2015.02.021.
27. Shaheen NJ, Weinberg DS, Denberg TD, Chou R, Qaseem A, Shekelle P. Upper endoscopy for gastroesophageal reflux disease: best practice advice from the clinical guidelines committee of the American College of Physicians. Ann Intern Med. 2012;157(11):808–16. https://doi. org/10.7326/0003-4819-157-11-201212040-00008.
28. Kahrilas PJ, Shaheen NJ, Vaezi MF, Hiltz SW, Black E, Modlin IM, et al. American Gastroenterological Association Medical Position Statement on the management of gastro-esophageal reflux disease. Gastroenterology. 2008;135(4):1383–91, 91.e1-5. https://doi. org/10.1053/j.gastro.2008.08.045.
29. DeVault KR, Castell DO, American College of G. Updated guidelines for the diagnosis and treatment of gastroesophageal reflux disease. Am J Gastroenterol. 2005;100(1):190–200. https://doi.org/10.1111/j.1572-0241.2005.41217.x.
30. Shaheen NJ, Falk GW, Iyer PG, Gerson LB, American College of G. ACG clinical guideline: diagnosis and management of Barrett's esophagus. Am J Gastroenterol. 2016;111(1):30–50; quiz 1. https://doi.org/10.1038/ajg.2015.322.
31. Hanna S, Rastogi A, Weston AP, Totta F, Schmitz R, Mathur S, et al. Detection of Barrett's esoph-agus after endoscopic healing of erosive esophagitis. Am J Gastroenterol. 2006;101(7):1416–20. https://doi.org/10.1111/j.1572-0241.2006.00631.x.
32. Roman S, Gyawali CP, Savarino E, Yadlapati R, Zerbib F, Wu J, et al. Ambulatory reflux monitoring for diagnosis of gastro-esophageal reflux disease: update of the Porto consen-sus and recommendations from an international consensus group. Neurogastroenterol Motil. 2017;29(10):1–15. https://doi.org/10.1111/nmo.13067.
33. Vaezi MF, Choksi Y. Mucosal impedance: a new way to diagnose reflux disease and how it could change your practice. Am J Gastroenterol. 2017;112(1):4–7. https://doi.org/10.1038/ ajg.2016.513.
34. Ward MA, Dunst CM, Teitelbaum EN, Halpin VJ, Reavis KM, Swanstrom LL, et al. Impedance-pH monitoring on medications does not reliably confirm the presence of gas-troesophageal reflux disease in patients referred for antireflux surgery. Surg Endosc. 2018;32(2):889–94. https://doi.org/10.1007/s00464-017-5759-7.
35. Hirano I, Zhang Q, Pandolfino JE, Kahrilas PJ. Four-day bravo pH capsule monitoring with and without proton pump inhibitor therapy. Clin Gastroenterol Hepatol. 2005;3(11):1083–8.
36. Ates F, Yuksel ES, Higginbotham T, Slaughter JC, Mabary J, Kavitt RT, et al. Mucosal imped-ance discriminates GERD from non-GERD conditions. Gastroenterology. 2015;148(2):334–43. https://doi.org/10.1053/j.gastro.2014.10.010.
37. Ness-Jensen E, Hveem K, El-Serag H, Lagergren J. Lifestyle intervention in gastroesophageal reflux disease. Clin Gastroenterol Hepatol. 2016;14(2):175–82 e1-3. https://doi.org/10.1016/j. cgh.2015.04.176.
38. Phupong V, Hanprasertpong T. Interventions for heartburn in pregnancy. Cochrane Database Syst Rev. 2015;19(9):CD011379. https://doi.org/10.1002/14651858.CD011379.pub2.
39. De Ruigh A, Roman S, Chen J, Pandolfino JE, Kahrilas PJ. Gaviscon double action liquid (antacid & alginate) is more effective than antacid in controlling post-prandial oesophageal acid exposure in GERD patients: a double-blind crossover study. Aliment Pharmacol Ther. 2014;40(5):531–7. https://doi.org/10.1111/apt.12857.
40. Leiman DA, Riff BP, Morgan S, Metz DC, Falk GW, French B, et al. Alginate therapy is effec-tive treatment for GERD symptoms: a systematic review and meta-analysis. Dis Esophagus. 2017;30(5):1–9. https://doi.org/10.1093/dote/dow020.
41. Wolfe MM, Sachs G. Acid suppression: optimizing therapy for gastroduodenal ulcer heal-ing, gastroesophageal reflux disease, and stress-related erosive syndrome. Gastroenterology. 2000;118(2):S9–S31. https://doi.org/10.1016/S0016-5085(00)70004-7.
42. Mainie I, Tutuian R, Castell DO. Addition of a H_2 receptor antagonist to PPI improves acid control and decreases nocturnal acid breakthrough. J Clin Gastroenterol. 2008;42(6):676–9. https://doi.org/10.1097/MCG.0b013e31814a4e5c.

43. Komazawa Y, Adachi K, Mihara T, Ono M, Kawamura A, Fujishiro H, et al. Tolerance to famotidine and ranitidine treatment after 14 days of administration in healthy subjects without helicobacter pylori infection. J Gastroenterol Hepatol. 2003;18(6):678–82.
44. Fackler WK, Ours TM, Vaezi MF, Richter JE. Long-term effect of H2RA therapy on nocturnal gastric acid breakthrough. Gastroenterology. 2002;122(3):625–32.
45. Kahrilas PJ. Gastroesophageal reflux disease. JAMA. 1996;276(12):983–8. https://doi.org/10.1001/jama.1996.03540120061035.
46. Xue S, Katz PO, Banerjee P, Tutuian R, Castell DO. Bedtime H2 blockers improve nocturnal gastric acid control in GERD patients on proton pump inhibitors. Aliment Pharmacol Ther. 2001;15(9):1351–6.
47. Ours TM, Fackler WK, Richter JE, Vaezi MF. Nocturnal acid breakthrough: clinical significance and correlation with esophageal acid exposure. Am J Gastroenterol. 2003;98(3):545–50.
48. Hatlebakk JG, Katz PO, Camacho-Lobato L, Castell DO. Proton pump inhibitors: better acid suppression when taken before a meal than without a meal. Aliment Pharmacol Ther. 2000;14(10):1267–72.
49. Lee RD, Vakily M, Mulford D, Wu J, Atkinson SN. Clinical trial: the effect and timing of food on the pharmacokinetics and pharmacodynamics of dexlansoprazole MR, a novel dual delayed release formulation of a proton pump inhibitor--evidence for dosing flexibility. Aliment Pharmacol Ther. 2009;29(8):824–33. https://doi.org/10.1111/j.1365-2036.2009.03979.x.
50. Chowers Y, Atarot T, Pratha VS, Fass R. The effect of once daily omeprazole and succinic acid (VECAM) vs once daily omeprazole on 24-h intragastric pH. Neurogastroenterol Motil. 2012;24(5):426–31, e208-9. https://doi.org/10.1111/j.1365-2982.2012.01884.x.
51. Chiba N, De Gara CJ, Wilkinson JM, Hunt RH. Speed of healing and symptom relief in grade II to IV gastroesophageal reflux disease: a meta-analysis. Gastroenterology. 1997;112(6):1798–810.
52. Sigterman KE, van Pinxteren B, Bonis PA, Lau J, Numans ME. Short-term treatment with proton pump inhibitors, H2-receptor antagonists and prokinetics for gastro-oesophageal reflux disease-like symptoms and endoscopy negative reflux disease. Cochrane Database Syst Rev. 2013;31(5):CD002095. https://doi.org/10.1002/14651858.CD002095.pub5.
53. Kirchheiner J, Glatt S, Fuhr U, Klotz U, Meineke I, Seufferlein T, et al. Relative potency of proton-pump inhibitors-comparison of effects on intragastric pH. Eur J Clin Pharmacol. 2009;65(1):19–31. https://doi.org/10.1007/s00228-008-0576-5.
54. Gralnek IM, Dulai GS, Fennerty MB, Spiegel BM. Esomeprazole versus other proton pump inhibitors in erosive esophagitis: a meta-analysis of randomized clinical trials. Clin Gastroenterol Hepatol. 2006;4(12):1452–8. https://doi.org/10.1016/j.cgh.2006.09.013.
55. Ip S, Chung M, Moorthy D, Yu WW, Lee J, Chan JA, et al. AHRQ comparative effectiveness reviews. Comparative effectiveness of management strategies for gastroesophageal reflux disease: update. Rockville, MD: Agency for Healthcare Research and Quality (US); 2011.
56. Wu MS, Tan SC, Xiong T. Indirect comparison of randomised controlled trials: comparative efficacy of dexlansoprazole vs. esomeprazole in the treatment of gastro-oesophageal reflux disease. Aliment Pharmacol Ther. 2013;38(2):190–201. https://doi.org/10.1111/apt.12349.
57. Shin JM, Sachs G. Pharmacology of proton pump inhibitors. Curr Gastroenterol Rep. 2008;10(6):528–34.
58. Freedberg DE, Kim LS, Yang YX. The risks and benefits of long-term use of proton pump inhibitors: expert review and best practice advice from the American Gastroenterological Association. Gastroenterology. 2017;152(4):706–15. https://doi.org/10.1053/j.gastro.2017.01.031.
59. Yadlapati R, Kahrilas PJ. When is proton pump inhibitor use appropriate? BMC Med. 2017;15(1):36. https://doi.org/10.1186/s12916-017-0804-x.
60. Yamashita H, Kanamori A, Kano C, Hashimura H, Matsumoto K, Tsujimae M, et al. The effects of switching to vonoprazan, a novel potassium-competitive acid blocker, on gastric acidity and reflux patterns in patients with erosive esophagitis refractory to proton pump inhibitors. Digestion. 2017;96(1):52–9. https://doi.org/10.1159/000478255.
61. Savarino E, Martinucci I, Furnari M, Romana C, Pellegatta G, Moscatelli A et al. Vonoprazan for treatment of gastroesophageal reflux: pharmacodynamic and pharmacokinetic consider-

ations. Expert Opin Drug Metab Toxicol. 2016:1–9. doi:https://doi.org/10.1080/17425255.20 16.1214714.

62. Baldi F. PPI-refractory GERD: an intriguing, probably overestimated, phenomenon. Curr Gastroenterol Rep. 2015;17(7):451. https://doi.org/10.1007/s11894-015-0451-3.

63. Gunaratnam NT, Jessup TP, Inadomi J, Lascewski DP. Sub-optimal proton pump inhibitor dosing is prevalent in patients with poorly controlled gastro-oesophageal reflux disease. Aliment Pharmacol Ther. 2006;23(10):1473–7. https://doi.org/10.1111/j.1365-2036.2006.02911.x.

64. Fass R, Gasiorowska A. Refractory GERD: what is it? Curr Gastroenterol Rep. 2008;10(3):252–7.

Approach to Patients with Esophageal Dysphagia

2

Steven P. Bowers

Introduction

Dysphagia refers to the subjective sense that swallowing is impeded or hindered. Population studies have suggested that 16% of a Western population (Australia) has sensed this at some point over a lifetime [1]. Although the prevalence of dysphagia increases with age, it should not be attributed to a normal consequence of aging. Dysphagia can occur acutely and require immediate treatment, can be of insidious onset and progressive, or may occur chronically in paroxysms. Dysphagia is the presenting symptom of a wide range of disorders ranging from locally advanced foregut cancer, to connective tissue disorders, to benign and idiopathic gut functional disorders. Because of the consequences of delaying the diagnosis of a potentially treatable disorder or malignancy, dysphagia is an alarm symptom that cannot be ignored and must be investigated. This chapter will detail the evaluation and etiology of the symptom of esophageal dysphagia.

Presentation

Esophageal dysphagia should be considered separately from globus sensation, the sensation that there is an object remaining in the hypopharynx between meals, and odynophagia, pain with swallowing. The primary focus of the initial interview with the patient should be to determine if the dysphagia is of esophageal origin, or oropharyngeal origin. Oropharyngeal dysphagia relates to difficulty initiating a swallow in the oral preparatory phase or hypopharyngeal phase of swallowing, and generally occurs immediately on swallowing, and is associated with coughing, the sense of choking, or nasal regurgitation. Oropharyngeal dysphagia should be

S. P. Bowers, M.D.
Davis 3N Surgery, Mayo Clinic Florida, Jacksonville, FL, USA
e-mail: bowers.steven@mayo.edu

© Springer International Publishing AG, part of Springer Nature 2018
D. Oleynikov, P. M. Fisichella (eds.), *A Mastery Approach to Complex Esophageal Diseases*, https://doi.org/10.1007/978-3-319-75795-7_2

considered separately. Although some general patterns have been observed in patients presenting with esophageal dysphagia, analysis of symptoms alone is never sufficient to classify the cause of dysphagia. However, assessment of the quality of dysphagia may serve as a lead point to investigation.

Acute Dysphagia

Patients presenting with acute dysphagia may present to the emergency room. Because the esophagus is so sensitive to stretch, patients with an impacted food bolus are compelled to seek emergency treatment. Such patients may complain of needing to regurgitate and expectorate their swallowed saliva, and are aware that a food bolus has not passed into the stomach. Treatment is with immediate upper flexible endoscopy, with or without a trial of intravenous glucagon, with retrieval of the bolus or assisted transit of the bolus into the stomach. Patients presenting with a first time food bolus impaction and no prior history of dysphagia are most likely to have eosinophilic esophagitis or peptic esophageal stricture due to gastroesophageal reflux (GERD) as the etiology [2].

Chronic Dysphagia

Sensation in the esophagus is such that patients may have symptoms referred more proximally in their esophagus, but rarely will symptoms be referred distally [3, 4]. Therefore, patients presenting with discomfort in their upper thoracic or cervical esophagus may have causative pathology in any aspect of the esophagus, proximal or distal. But patients presenting with symptoms of dysphagia of the lower thoracic or distal esophagus will usually have pathology at the distal esophagus or gastroesophageal junction (GEJ).

Patients can usually discriminate whether dysphagia occurs stereotypically with a certain size bolus of food, and whether dysphagia occurs with solids or liquids or both. Generally, dysphagia to only solids implies there is a mechanical obstruction, whereas, dysphagia to solids and liquids implies an esophageal motility disorder is associated with the symptoms. Dysphagia to all solids implies a high-grade esophageal obstruction.

Patients with chronic dysphagia have usually made lifestyle and dietary changes to avoid the discomfort of dysphagia, and although weight loss is often observed with solid food dysphagia, paradoxical weight gain can occur with a change to softer high energy density foods. Dysphagia in the setting of a history of smoking and binge drinking should alert the clinician to a higher suspicion of squamous cancer of the esophagus. Dysphagia in the setting of long history of GERD should similarly raise suspicion for adenocarcinoma of the distal esophagus. However, one third of patients found to have esophageal adenocarcinoma have no history of reflux symptoms, and 40% of patients found to have achalasia have symptoms initially attributed to GERD [5]. Associated muscle weakness with dysphagia should raise suspicion for neuromuscular diseases that may also have associated oropharyngeal swallowing disorders: ALS, polymyositis, and muscular dystrophy. And the association of connective tissue disorders with dysphagia prompts thoughts of scleroderma esophagus. Because the specificity of symptoms associations with dysphagia is so poor, further testing is required in all patients with dysphagia.

Diagnostic Testing

Contrast Esophagram

Contrast esophagram and upper flexible endoscopy (EGD) are complementary tests in the assessment of the patients with dysphagia. It has been customary teaching to have patients undergo Barium esophagram as the initial test, because knowledge of anatomical derangements found at barium swallow (Zenker's diverticulum, proximal esophageal webs and esophageal tumors or rings) may facilitate EGD or enable biopsy or treatment at the initial EGD session [6]. Barium swallow is the definitive test to identify paraesophageal hernia as the etiology of dysphagia and the most sensitive test to identify esophageal webs or rings.

Prone esophagram allows greater sensitivity in detecting subtle esophageal rings, and air contrast barium swallow may detect mucosal irregularity for future biopsy. Barium swallow with 13 mm barium tablet or barium soaked marshmallow is helpful in detecting an abnormality in solid bolus transport or mechanical obstruction of the esophagus. In patients known or suspected of having esophageal achalasia, a timed barium swallow is done by measuring the column of barium at 1, 2 and 5 min after swallowing liquid barium. This is primarily helpful in measuring progress after a procedure to improve esophageal emptying.

Upper Flexible Endoscopy—EGD

EGD is the first line test with the greatest yield in the evaluation of dysphagia and allows mucosal biopsy for the identification of Barrett's esophagus and esophageal cancer, as well as eosinophilic esophagitis. In patients with dysphagia undergoing EGD, routine biopsy should be performed in all patients, including at least four total biopsies of one proximal and one distal site down the esophageal lumen. Due to the ease and safety of through-the-scope dilation, empiric dilation of the LES should additionally be considered in patients with dysphagia. EGD is the standard for identifying or ruling out mucosal abnormalities, but is not a sensitive test for the identification of esophageal motility disorders.

Esophageal Motility Testing

High-resolution manometry and use of the Chicago classification scheme [7] to identify esophageal motility disorders has standardized the classification of esophageal motility patterns into major disorders which are always associated with

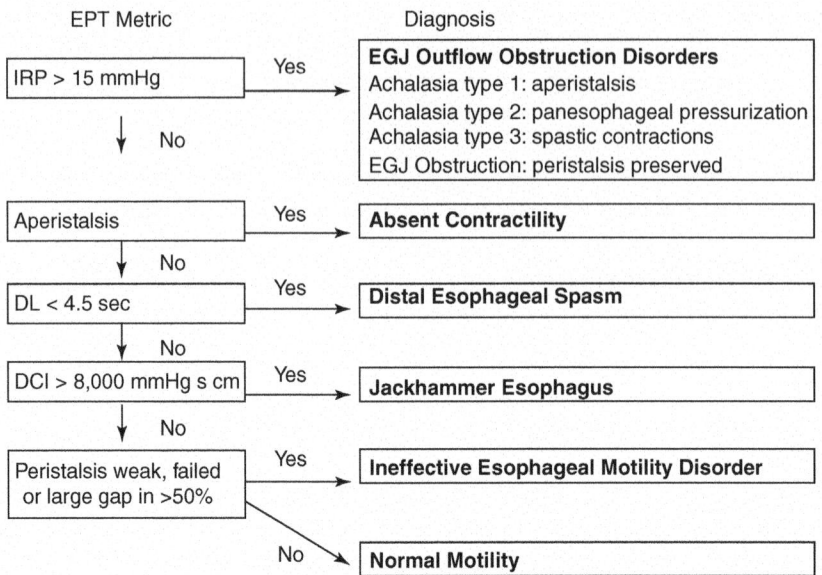

EPT Metric   Diagnosis

Fig. 2.1 Chicago Classification version 3. The hierarchical algorithm of the Chicago Classification is represented here, developed by the International High Resolution Manometry Working Group [8]. Abbreviations: *IRP* integrated relaxation pressure, *DL* distal latency, *DCI* distal contractile integral

symptoms. The prioritization of the Chicago classification scheme is to first identify the variants of esophageal achalasia, then to identify the other major hypermotile and hypomotile esophageal motility disorders, and finally to identify minor motility disorders [7]. Figure 2.1 diagrams the diagnostic algorithm of the Chicago Classification version 3. In those patients found to have no structural cause for dysphagia on contrast esophagram or endoscopy, motility testing identifies a causative motility disorder in 50% of patients [9].

Analysis of high-resolution manometry is performed in a systematic fashion, with the patients swallowing ten times of a 5 mL bolus of fluid. Initial assessment is of the completeness of each attempted swallow. For each complete swallow, five key metrics are measured from the esophageal topography plot (EPT). The first is the integrated relaxation pressure (IRP), measured as the mean nadir pressure of the lower esophageal sphincter (LES) in a 4 s time after swallow is initiated. This value establishes the presence or absence of achalasia variants, based on the associated findings of peristalsis, esophageal pressurization or spastic contractions.

Next, the time from initiation of swallowing to the slowing of the peristaltic wave at the esophageal ampulla (the contractile deceleration point, or CDP) is termed the distal latency (DL). This value establishes the premature- or simultaneous-nature of the peristaltic wave and is the metric used to diagnose distal esophageal spasm. The amplitude of esophageal peristalsis is measured as the integrated volume of the esophageal pressure topography map and is defined as the distal contractile integral

(DCI). The DCI metric defines both hypermotile major motility disorders (jackhammer esophagus) and minor hypomotility disorders (ineffective esophageal motility disorder). The slope of the peristaltic wave through the esophageal body is defined as the contractile front velocity (CFV) and is used as the metric to measure the rapidity of the peristaltic wave, a metric which no longer is associated with a named motility disorder. Finally, the length of any gap in the 20 mmHg isobaric curve on the peristaltic wave is measured, with a 5 cm gap signifying a fractured peristaltic wave. Simultaneous esophageal impedance testing is able to associate minor motility disturbances with incomplete esophageal emptying.

Other Diagnostic Modalities

When EGD is suspicious for vascular malformations impinging on the esophagus, a condition called dysphagia lusoria, CT scan of the chest is beneficial. Retroesophageal right subclavian artery is the most common of these malformations, but is generally asymptomatic. Impedance planimetry is used as an adjunctive test to measure esophageal compliance and can monitor progress in treating esophageal achalasia and eosinophilic esophagitis.

Differential Diagnosis of Esophageal Dysphagia

GERD Related Dysphagia

Reflux disease can be the cause of both structural- and motility-origin dysphagia and is by a considerable margin the most common cause of dysphagia. Peptic esophageal stricture is more common in elderly male patients with long reflux history, but is found in up to 10% of all patients undergoing endoscopy for evaluation of reflux symptoms. Peptic strictures occur most commonly at the squamo-columnar junction in the form of Schatzki's ring. Meat impaction is common, approaching an incidence of 13 per 100,000 population per year [10]. Short term treatment is by esophageal dilation, but long term treatment by decreasing GERD, including by antireflux surgery, reduces the incidence of repeat dilation [11].

Reflux also causes dysphagia by mechanism of ineffective esophageal motility induced by esophagitis. Gastroesophageal reflux disease is associated with hypocontractile states and GERD is likely causative of impaired peristalsis and decreased peristaltic amplitude. Hypotensive LES and inappropriate LES relaxation are similarly causative of GERD, and ineffective motility further exacerbates reflux by mechanism of delayed esophageal clearance.

Ineffective esophageal motility disorder (IEMD) is defined by the Chicago classification as greater than 50% of peristaltic waves that are failed, weak or have large gaps, but this definition does not accurately describe patients with IEMD with dysphagia [12]. As measured by HRM and a prior version of the Chicago classification, weak peristalsis has shown a higher correlation with dysphagia than frequent failed peristalsis, but these disorders are considered together as a minor disorder because there are considerable numbers of healthy individuals who exhibit these findings.

With intensive antireflux therapy, IEMD may improve, but rarely normalizes. With antireflux surgery, partial fundoplication is associated with greater improvement in IEMD than total fundoplication and greater relief of IEMD associated dysphagia [13, 14]. Regarding surgical decision making in patients with IEMD seeking antireflux operations, it is the author's practice to consider whether the degree of IEMD is proportionate to the severity of GERD, based on degree of erosive esophagitis and pH testing. When peristaltic failure and/or dysphagia are out of proportion to the level of GERD, partial fundoplication is recommended.

Patients with aperistalsis thought due to severe GERD, without any findings consistent with connective tissue disorder, may be treated intensively with proton pump inhibitor therapy for 3–4 months and a motility study repeated. If there is significant improvement in esophageal peristalsis, then Nissen fundoplication can be considered.

Post-surgical Dysphagia

All patients undergoing fundoplication will experience immediate post-operative dysphagia related to edema of the operative site, and it is incumbent on the surgical team to prepare the patient's dietary expectations accordingly. Patients after Nissen fundoplication are usually able to return to solid food diet in a 4–8 week window after operation. However, approximately 5–10% of patients after Nissen fundoplication will be expected to struggle with the return to a solid diet. Aerophagia and early post-operative dry heaving increase post-operative dysphagia in patients otherwise expected to have routine recovery.

Postoperative dysphagia that does not improve by 8–12 weeks should be considered for esophageal dilation. This persistent postoperative dysphagia is associated with increased preoperative LES pressure and with incomplete preoperative LES relaxation [15]. Emerging use of multiple repetitive swallows during HRM has enabled some prediction of the "esophageal peristaltic reserve". When three small swallows are made in short succession, there is inhibition of esophageal body peristalsis and LES tone; this is followed in the normal state by an augmented esophageal contraction. The ratio of the DCI of the augmented contraction, relative to the average of the ten prior swallows, has predictive value for the absence of post-fundoplication dysphagia [8].

Patients undergoing magnetic sphincter augmentation are expected to experience dysphagia in the second to fourth week of recovery corresponding to the time period of maximally dense postoperative adhesive disease following operation. It is imperative that these patients persist on a solid or semi-solid diet through this period to prevent fibrotic adhesions from fusing some of the magnetic beads together. Antispasmotic medications, steroids, or even esophageal dilation can be required in this time period.

There are a small number of patients who develop worsening esophageal peristalsis after antireflux operation. When associated with hiatal stenosis or failure to pass a 13 mm barium tablet, aperistalsis in this setting can be indistinguishable from an achalasia variant. Failing esophageal dilation, remedial operation may be required to remove any foreign material at the hiatus and convert to partial fundoplication, with or without Heller myotomy.

Bariatric operations induce restriction of the upper stomach by creating stenosis via stapling (Roux en Y gastric bypass and sleeve resection of the stomach) or by extrinsic compression (adjustable gastric band). Dysphagia is not uncommon after adjustable gastric band and when associated with esophageal dilation or pouch enlargement would indicate band explant. Dysphagia can result from several different mechanisms after sleeve gastrectomy: a tight sleeve may create excessive restriction, disruption of gastric sling fibers with cardia stapling may induce spastic motility disorder, transhiatal herniation of the upper sleeve may create tortuosity of the distal esophagus, or uncontrolled GERD may induce IEMD. Although esophageal dilation for early postoperative sleeve-related dysphagia may be helpful for stenosis of the upper stomach, remedial operation with conversion to Roux en Y gastric bypass is often the best course of action.

Esophageal Cancer

Despite knowledge of the association between GERD and Barrett's esophagus and its progression to esophageal adenocarcinoma, and increasing proportion of citizens taking prescription proton pump inhibitors, the incidence of esophageal adenocarcinoma continues to increase in Western civilization. Adenocarcinomas of the gastroesophageal junction and cardia may be associated with an achalasia-like syndrome, pseudoachalasia, that be require endoscopic ultrasound to distinguish from achalasia. New onset dysphagia and rapid weight loss generally implies at least locally invasive disease that is not amenable to endoscopic resection. While long-term survival with chemo-radiation and subsequent resection has been shown to approach 50%, the overall prognosis remains dire for adenocarcinoma of the esophagus. Squamous cancer of the esophagus presents generally in the proximal to mid esophagus, is more radiation sensitive with approximately double the rate of complete response to chemoradiation, and has a higher likelihood of survival with multimodality therapy [16].

Esophageal Strictures

Approximately 75% of esophageal strictures are reflux related. These are typically passable by an endoscope, located at the squamo-columnar line, and short. Such strictures can be dilated by either freely-passed, weighted Maloney dilators, plastic Savary-Guillard over the wire bougies, or hydrostatic through-the-scope dilators. The effectiveness is based on clinician experience and generally thought to be equivalent. Relief from dysphagia occurs with dilation to greater than 13 mm, but longer relief of dysphagia is associated with dilation to 16 mm or greater [17]. It is customary to start at the estimated stricture diameter and to dilate no more than 2 mm per session. Repeat dilation sessions approximately one-week apart may be required to achieve successful relief of dysphagia. Patients should be placed on twice daily proton pump inhibitor therapy for up to 1 year after stricture dilation, and GERD symptom control correlates with freedom from stricture recurrence [18].

Refractory or complicated strictures may require additional endoscopic techniques for successful dilation. In order of increasing invasiveness, additional techniques include: injection into the stricture of the steroid triamcinolone prior to dilation, endoscopic radial incision or biopsy of the stricture to break the mucosal ring, or placement of an expandable plastic, biodegradable, or dog-bone shaped flanged and covered metallic stent. Stents should be removed after 6–8 weeks and the stricture reassessed. An algorithm of progressive therapies for refractory strictures has not been systematically studied.

Non-peptic strictures make up the minority of esophageal strictures but account for a greater percentage of complicated strictures. Definitive chemo-radiation therapy has been proven effective for patients with squamous cancer of the esophagus exhibiting a complete pathological response to therapy; however, radiation-induced stricture is a not infrequent result of this therapy. Mucosa-limited esophageal adenocarcinoma may be treated with endoscopic mucosal dissection/resection with favorable recurrence free survival, but circumferential or near-circumferential resection is associated with up to 45% rate of esophageal stricture [19]. Other causes of non-peptic stricture include toxic ingestions of liquids such as lye. Esophageal anastomotic strictures occurring early after operation may be associated with leak, ischemia or fistula and stenting is preferable in such cases.

Esophageal Motility Disorders

With the exception of esophageal achalasia and scleroderma esophagus, disorders associated with distinct pathologic findings designating them as disease processes, all esophageal motility disorders are defined in terms of their metrics on high resolution manometry and by the current classification by the Chicago Classification v3.0.

Esophageal Achalasia

Esophageal achalasia is a disease characterized by esophageal outflow obstruction (caused by inadequate relaxation of the LES) and a pressurized and/or dilated esophagus with nonprogressive swallow responses. In achalasia, there is degeneration of ganglion cells in the myenteric plexus of the esophageal wall, related to absence in the LES of the neurotransmitters nitric oxide and vasoactive intestinal polypeptide [20]. Experimental models have long suggested that the peristaltic abnormalities seen in esophageal achalasia are secondary to the outflow obstruction [21]. However, by the water-perfused manometry study and standard motility classification, aperistalsis was used as the most important motility abnormality identified in achalasia. Use of high-resolution manometry studies and the Chicago classification have redirected the diagnosis to reflect the pathophysiologic findings of achalasia [8]. Esophageal achalasia had previously been classified into subtypes, classic and vigorous achalasia, based on the finding in the esophageal body, of vigorous repetitive and high-amplitude swallow responses. This classification had no clinical significance, however.

The Chicago classification has refined the subclassification of achalasia into subtypes based on the finding of esophageal pressurization and premature contractions [22–24]. With type 1 representing classic achalasia and type 2 identifying patients with panesophageal pressurization (to >30 mm Hg) in 20% or greater swallows. Type 3, or spastic achalasia identifies patients who have no intact peristalsis but have the finding, in 20% or greater swallows, of premature or simultaneous contractions (with DL < 4.5 s). Further, type 3 achalasia represents patients who may have been, by classical definitions, been diagnosed as having diffuse esophageal spasm with incomplete LES relaxation. These type 3 achalasia patients are more likely to present with chest pain as a prominent symptom. Of these subtypes, type 2 seems to be slightly more common than type 1, and type 3 is infrequent in most reported series.

Additionally, the Chicago classification has allowed for the identification of patients with an achalasia variant, with the finding of incompletely- or non-relaxing LES and some preservation of peristalsis [25]. The classification EGJ (esophagogastric junction) relaxation abnormality includes patients who are found on later study to have achalasia with aperistalsis, as well as those with pseudoachalasia and postoperative (postfundoplication) states.

The development of high-resolution manometry and the Chicago classification has both broadened and simplified the definitions of achalasia and its subtypes. Additionally, the Chicago classification subtypes have some added prognostic value that may aid in the formulation of surgical planning. Type 1 achalasia seems to have better outcomes with myotomy as the initial treatment when compared with endoscopic therapies (botulinum toxin injection or pneumatic balloon dilation) [22]. Type 2 achalasia seems to have the best outcomes regardless of the initial treatment strategy and type 3 has the worst outcomes irrespective of treatment strategy (botulinum toxin, pneumatic dilation, and myotomy). Based on the reported improved response of type 2 patients to any initial treatment, there may be greater support among gastroenterologists for initial endoscopic therapy in type 2 achalasia patients, with myotomy relegated to treatment failures in type 2 patients. However, because there is a spectrum of continuity between type 1 cases with pressurization to just below 30 mm Hg and type 2 cases, and marginal differences between type 3 cases and some achalasia variants, it is unrealistic to make a firm algorithm regarding treatment based strictly on achalasia sub-types.

Although laparoscopic Heller myotomy with partial fundoplication is accessible to most patients with achalasia in North America, the diffusion of centers offering peroral endoscopic myotomy (POEM) as a definitive treatment of achalasia has made this an option for most regions [26]. Because POEM is reflexogenic in one-third of patients without hiatal hernia, the presence of a hiatal hernia should be seen as a relative contraindication for the POEM procedure [27]. Otherwise, analysis of the outcomes for POEM based on reports from high-volume centers and the growing international experience essentially equates POEM outcomes with surgical myotomy without fundoplication by other approach [27–30].

Esophageal pulsion-type diverticula represent one of the most rare manifestations of achalasia, occurring in the author's experience in fewer than 5% of patients with achalasia. Although treatment of the underlying motility disorder yields acceptable results in most patients, the optimal surgical approach includes stapled diverticulectomy guided by intraoperative endoscopy, with Heller myotomy and partial fundoplication.

Hypercontractility States

Symptoms of dysphagia and chest pain are clinical scenarios that are suspicious for hypercontractile esophageal motility disorders. Although contrast esophagram may confirm a hypercontractile esophageal motility disorder, it is not sensitive enough to be used as a screening test. An esophageal motility study is required to establish a diagnosis and initiate treatment. Based on the Chicago classification and analysis of high-resolution manometry EPT metrics, there are two identified major hypercontractile abnormalities that are always associated with patient symptoms and never identified in normal individuals [31]. Using the new classification scheme, the number of patients diagnosed with hypercontractile motility disorders is markedly reduced and, because the most extreme cases have been selected, response to medications and natural history of the disorders as currently diagnosed are unknown.

Distal Esophageal Spasm

The name diffuse esophageal spasm has been something of a misnomer because it is the distal esophagus that is spastic [32]. DES is now the preferred terminology but both are used interchangeably. Patients with DES commonly present with dysphagia. Because of the observed response in DES patients to nitroglycerin, it is thought that DES may be pathophysiologically linked to a defect in esophageal nitric oxide production [33, 34]. Contrast esophagram may demonstrate the classic corkscrew esophagus or rosary bead esophagus; however, a normal contrast esophagram does not exclude DES. The hallmark of DES by classic esophageal motility study has been the finding of frequent simultaneous peristalsis. Classically, in one-third of patients there has been some abnormality of the LES (either hypertensive LES or incompletely relaxing LES) [35, 36]. However, with high-resolution manometry and interpreted by the Chicago classification, some of these latter patients would be now considered to have type 3 achalasia or an achalasia variant.

High-resolution manometry diagnostic criteria rely on measurement of DL to determine whether a peristaltic contraction is considered premature or simultaneous (DL < 4.5 s). The Chicago classification designates DES as having 20% or greater of swallows with DL less than 4.5 s. This is in contrast to the characteristic manometry finding of high-velocity peristalsis (CFV > 8–9 cm/s) to identify simultaneous contractions, or the findings of repetitive contractions or contractions of long duration (>6 s) in greater than 20% of peristaltic waves that previously constituted DES. The Chicago classification requires that there also be normal LES relaxation to distinguish DES from achalasia variants. Greater than two-thirds of patients previously diagnosed as having DES will now receive a different diagnosis using the Chicago classification [37]. Rapid contraction, defined as 20% or greater swallows with CFV greater than 9 cm/s was considered borderline motility by the Chicago classification version 2 [38] but is not considered an abnormality on the current classification.

Although patients with classically defined DES followed longitudinally show that the majority improve somewhat with time without directed medical therapy, [39] there are several classes of medication that have proven to be somewhat helpful in managing the disorder. The antidepressants trazodone and imipramine were found to decrease chest pain with DES, likely by modifying esophageal sensitivity [40, 41]. The phosphodiesterase inhibitor sildenafil has been associated with symptomatic relief [42]. Botulinum toxin delivered by endoscopic injection was found to decrease dysphagia [43].

The diagnostic criteria for DES are now more restrictive and DES now refers to a more distinct clinical phenotype. With the more restrictive definition, it should be infrequent that the surgeon encounters a patient with documented GERD and DES. In a patient with documented GERD who has diagnostic criteria for DES on preoperative high-resolution manometry, the surgeon should reassess which symptoms may be due to DES and, therefore, unlikely to respond to antireflux therapy. For patients with GERD who have prominent dysphagia symptoms and DES, Nissen fundoplication is not recommended. In patients with noncardiac chest pain found to have DES and GERD that are failing medical therapy, the surgeon should consider starting an antidepressant before or after antireflux surgery.

More commonly, the surgeon encounters patients who previously would have been diagnosed with DES but are now classified as having a nonspecific spastic motility disorder because of rapid or simultaneous contractions not fulfilling criteria for DES. Expectations should be revisited as to which symptoms are likely to improve after operation. In patients presenting with DES and refractory symptoms of dysphagia and chest pain, it is reasonable to perform endoscopic botulinum toxin injection. Although there are reported small series of POEM procedure for DES [29, 44], this should be viewed with caution because of the propensity for classically defined DES symptoms to lessen over time without intervention.

Jackhammer Esophagus

The hypercontractile esophagus is characterized by high-amplitude esophageal body peristaltic contractions, associated with chest pain and/or dysphagia. Using the water-perfused manometry system, the criteria for defining the disorder as nutcracker esophagus had undergone some evolution to a higher mean amplitude (from 180 to 220 mm Hg) to decrease the number of patients diagnosed with the disorder who had reflux symptoms rather than chest pain [45]. Using the high-resolution manometry system, the Chicago classification developed an entirely new metric, the DCI, and identified the threshold for which a single swallow with elevated DCI was always associated with dysphagia (DCI > 8000 mm Hg/cm/s), and termed this disorder jackhammer esophagus. This is reflective of the finding of repetitive contractions in most spastic hypercontractile waves. Mean DCI greater than 5000 mm Hg/cm/s based on ten swallows was termed hypertensive peristalsis; however, this finding is no longer considered abnormal.

The pathophysiology of the hypercontractile esophageal disorders is thought to be due to asynchrony in the circular and longitudinal smooth muscle of the esophagus during contraction. Because this is reversible with atropine, it thought to be due, in part, to a hypercholinergic state [46]. Treatment of hypercontractile esophagus is similar to treatment of DES. Diltiazem was found to relieve chest pain in patients with nutcracker esophagus [47]. Sildenafil, trazodone, and imipramine have also been found to be helpful [40–42]. Based on the pathophysiology of the disorder, anticholinergic medications would be expected to have treatment benefit. Endoscopic botulinum toxin injection has a response rate greater than 70% and half of treated patients have, at least temporarily, complete relief of chest pain [48]. Failing medical therapy, patients with nutcracker esophagus with severe dysphagia may undergo Heller myotomy with good relief of dysphagia; however, relief of chest pain is less certain with laparoscopic Heller myotomy [49]. Small series of POEM for hypercontractile esophagus show promise, with high rates of relief of chest pain [29].

The classically described nutcracker esophagus has been associated with GERD. The finding of hypertensive peristalsis in a patient with GERD should not alter the treatment plan for antireflux surgery. Because jackhammer esophagus is a finding always associated with chest pain or dysphagia, the treatment plan should reflect the expectation that this disorder will not resolve with treatment of GERD and should be specifically addressed. However, definitive treatment studies have not been performed using these specific criteria for hypercontractile esophagus.

Hypocontractile States

There are distinct pathological findings associated with the esophageal manifestations of systemic sclerosis, or scleroderma. Scleroderma esophagus is caused by atrophy and sclerosis of the smooth muscle of the esophagus; the striated proximal esophageal muscle is spared. Thus scleroderma, mixed connective tissue disorders or collagen vascular diseases, with esophageal manifestations should be considered separately from ineffective esophageal motility associated with GERD. Scleroderma esophagus is defined as aperistalsis with low or absent LES pressure (resting pressure < 10 mm Hg). Esophageal findings are present in over 70% of patients with the typical skin manifestations of scleroderma [50, 51]. Esophageal manometry findings similar to that found in scleroderma and the mixed connective tissue disorders may be found in other diseases, such as polymyositis, dermatomyositis, muscular dystrophy and Sjogren's. Sjogren's syndrome is also associated with the symptoms of dysphagia, and xerostomia compounds the problem of esophageal dysmotility in these patients.

The primary consideration in managing scleroderma esophagus is preventing development of peptic esophageal stricture, malnutrition, or recurrent aspiration pneumonia. Although a loose Nissen fundoplication may be used [52], more recent reports recommend partial fundoplication [53], and consideration should be given to placement of gastrostomy tube for feeding access during antireflux surgery [54].

Functional Dysphagia

Functional dysphagia was characterized by the Rome III Consensus as one of four benign functional disorders of the esophagus, along with globus sensation, functional heartburn, and functional chest pain [55]. The criteria for diagnosis include presence of the symptom of dysphagia for at least 6 months, including the last 3 months, absence of evidence that GERD is associated by both upper flexible endoscopy, contrast esophagram, and esophageal physiologic testing, and absence of histopathology-based esophageal motility disorders. Emerging reports suggest that 25% of patients with functional dysphagia have subtle esophageal motility disorders such as incomplete LES relaxation or even delayed LES relaxation (over 50% of swallows with greater than 5 s between UES and LES relaxation) [56].

Treatment is by reduction of stress that may exacerbate the sensation of dysphagia [57], desensitization of the esophagus with tricyclic antidepressants or selective serotonin reuptake inhibitors. Upper flexible endoscopy with esophageal dilation may be utilized if the lower esophageal sphincter is found to be incompletely relaxing on high-resolution motility [55] or if barium tablet is delayed on contrast esophagram.

Eosinophilic Esophagitis

The classic presentation of eosinophilic esophagitis (EoE) is dysphagia in a young male with asthma, eczema or atopic disorders and history of prior esophageal meat impaction. EGD will identify in the majority one of the characteristic findings of edema, esophageal longitudinal furrows, trachealization of the esophagus with concentric rings, or exudates, but EGD may visually be normal in up to 25% of patients with biopsy proven eosinophilic esophagitis [58, 59]. Up to 15% of all patients undergoing EGD for evaluation of dysphagia will be found to have

EoE [60]. The diagnosis is based on the finding in esophageal biopsy of greater than 15 eosinophils per high power field in the squamous epithelium of the esophagus—in EoE, the eosinophils are limited to the esophagus and persist after a two-month trial of proton pump inhibitor to exclude reflux-related eosinophilia [59]. With at least four esophageal biopsies the sensitivity of detecting eosinophils reaches 98%. When EOE is suspected in the presence of other foregut symptoms, EGD should also include gastric and duodenal biopsies to document eosinophilic gastroenteritis.

Because EoE is an antigen-mediated cellular hypersensitivity disorder, allergy testing to reduce dietary allergens can be considered for therapy. Elimination diet of allergic foods can be based on allergy testing or empirically-empiric elimination diets are generally more effective. The foods that are known to elicit the greatest IgE response and are triggers of EoE are milk, eggs, legumes and wheat. Once successful response in esophageal eosinophilia is documented by endoscopic biopsy, foods can be reintroduced sequentially with repeat endoscopic guidance. Specific validated questionnaires (MDQ-30) may be used to assess the level of dysphagia due to EoE and to guide treatment [61].

In addition, swallowed topical steroids (budesonide) have been proven effective in reducing symptoms and maintaining remission from symptoms [62], but are not as effective in patients with esophageal stricture [63]. Endoscopic dilation has classically been described as having a higher risk of perforation in patients with untreated EoE-perforation has occurred even during diagnostic endoscopy in patients with EoE. Generally, dilation is reserved for EoE related rings or strictures who are failures of first-line medical therapy and should be performed cautiously.

Conclusion

Dysphagia is an alarm symptom that the clinician should seek to explain. Upper endoscopy has the highest yield in ruling out esophageal cancer, erosive esophagitis due to severe GERD, and eosinophilic esophagitis; and endoscopic dilation may provide immediate relief from rings and strictures. Contrast esophagram can detect subtle rings and a barium pill can detect delayed esophageal emptying due to paraesophageal hernia. Esophageal motility testing is essential for diagnosing major esophageal motility disorders, and emerging refinements of the high resolution manometry are improving the diagnosis of functional dysphagia and may be predictive of post-surgical dysphagia.

References

1. Eslick GD, Talley NJ. Dysphagia: epidemiology, risk factors and impact on quality of life–a population-based study. Aliment Pharmacol Ther. 2008;27:971–9.
2. Desai TK, Stecevic V, Chang CH, et al. Association of eosinophilic inflammation with esophageal food impaction in adults. Gastrointest Endosc. 2005;61:795.
3. Roeder BE, Murray JA, Dierkhising RA. Patient localization of esophageal dysphagia. Dig Dis Sci. 2004;49:697–701.

4. Wilcox CM, Alexander LN, Clark WS. Localization of an obstructing esophageal lesion. Is the patient accurate? Dig Dis Sci. 1995;40:2192.
5. Spechler SJ, Souza RF, Rosenberg SJ, et al. Heartburn in patients with achalasia. Gut. 1995;37:305.
6. American Gastroenterological Association medical position statement on management of oropharyngeal dysphagia. Gastroenterology. 1999;116:452.
7. Bowers SP. Esophageal motility disorders. Surg Clin North Am. 2015;95(3):467–82.
8. Kahrilas PJ, Bredenord AJ, Fox M, Gyawali CP, Roman S, Smout AJPM, Pandolfino JE, International High Resolution Manometry Working Group. The Chicago Clasification of esophageal motility disorders, v3.0. Neurogastroenterol Motil. 2015;27:160–74.
9. AJ DM Jr, Allen ML, Lynn RB, Zamani S. Clinical value of esophageal motility testing. Dig Dis. 1998;16:198.
10. Gretarsdottir HM, Jonasson JG, Björnsson ES. Etiology and management of esophageal food impaction: a population based study. Scand J Gastroenterol. 2015;50:513.
11. Spivak H, Farrell TM, Trus TL, Branum GD, Waring JP, Hunter JG. Laparoscopic fundoplication for dysphagia and peptic esophageal stricture. J Gastrointest Surg. 1998;2(6):555–60.
12. Tutuian R, Castell DO. Clarification of the esophageal function defect in patients with manometric ineffective esophageal motility: studies using combined impedance-manometry. Clin Gastroenterol Hepatol. 2004;2:230.
13. Fibbe C, Layer P, Keller J, et al. Esophageal motility in reflux disease before and after fundoplication: a prospective, randomized, clinical, and manometric study. Gastroenterology. 2001;121:5.
14. Strate U, Emmerman A, Fibbe C, et al. Laparoscopic fundoplication: Nissen versus Toupet two-year outcome of a prospective randomized study of 200 patients regarding preoperative esophageal motility. Surg Endosc. 2008;22:21–30.
15. Blom D, Peters JH, DeMeester TR, et al. Physiologic mechanism and preoperative prediction of new-onset dysphagia after laparoscopic Nissen fundoplication. J Gastrointest Surg. 2002;6(1):22–7.
16. Shapiro J, van Lanschot JJB, Hulshof MCCM, The CROSS Study Group, et al. Neoadjuvant chemoradiotherapy plus surgery versus surgery alone for oesophageal or junctional cancer (CROSS); long-term results of a randomized controlled trial. Lancet Oncol. 2015;16(9):1090–8.
17. van Halsema EE, Noordzij IC, van Berge Henegouwen MI, et al. Endoscopic dilation of benign esophageal anastomotic strictures over 16 mm has a longer lasting effect. Surg Endosc. 2017;31:1871.
18. Said A, Brust DJ, Gaumnitz EA, Reichelderfer M. Predictors of early recurrence of benign esophageal strictures. Am J Gastroenterol. 2003;98:1252.
19. Nagami Y, Shiba M, Ominami M, Sakai T, Minamoto H, Fukunaga S, Sugimori S, Tanaka F, Kamata N, Tanigawa T, Yamagami H, Watanabe T, Tominaga K, Fujiwara Y, Arakawa T. Single locoregional triamcinolone injection immediately after esophageal endoscopic submucosal dissection prevents stricture formation. Clin Transl Gastroenterol. 2017;23:8.
20. Ghoshal UC, Daschakraborty SB, Singh R. Pathogenesis of achalasia cardia. World J Gastroenterol. 2012;18(4):3050–7.
21. Khajanchee YS, VanAndel R, Jobe BA, et al. Electrical stimulation of the vagus nerve restores motility in an animal model of achalasia. J Gastrointest Surg. 2003;7(7):843–9.
22. Pandolfino JE, Kwiatek MA, Nealis T, et al. Achalasia: a new clinically relevant classification by high-resolution manometry. Gastroenterology. 2008;135:1526.
23. Salvador R, Costantini M, Zaninotto G, et al. The preoperative manometric pattern predicts the outcome of surgical treatment for esophageal achalasia. J Gastrointest Surg. 2010;14(11):1635–45.
24. Pratap N, Kalapala R, Darisetty S, et al. Achalasia cardia subtyping by high resolution manometry predicts the therapeutic outcome of pneumatic balloon dilatation. J Neurogastroenterol Motil. 2011;17(1):48–53.
25. Scherer JR, Kwiatek MA, Soper NJ, et al. Functional esophagogastric junction obstruction with intact peristalsis: a heterogeneous syndrome sometimes akin to achalasia. J Gastrointest Surg. 2009;13:2219.

26. Patti MG, Andolfino C, Bowers SP, Soper NJ. POEM vs laparoscopic heller myotomy and fundoplication: which is now the gold standard for treatment of achalasia? J Gastrointest Surg. 2017;21(2):207–14.
27. Sharata AM, Dunst CM, Pescarus R, et al. Peroral endoscopic myotomy (POEM) for esophageal primary motility disorders: analysis of 100 consecutive patients. J Gastrointest Surg. 2015;19:161–70.
28. Inoue H, Tianle KM, Ikeda H, et al. Peroral endoscopic myotomy for esophageal achalasia: technique, indication and outcomes. Thorac Surg Clin. 2011;21(4):519–25.
29. Ling TS, Guo HM, Yang T, et al. Effectiveness of peroral endoscopic myotomy in the treatment of achalasia: a pilot trial in Chinese Han population with a minimum of one-year follow-up. J Dig Dis. 2014;15(7):352–8.
30. Von Renteln D, Fuchs KH, Breithaupt W, et al. Peroral endoscopic myotomy for the treatment of esophageal achalasia: an international multicenter study. Gastroenterology. 2013;145(2):309–11.
31. Roman S, Pandolfino JE, Chen J, et al. Phenotypes and clinical context of hypercontractility in high-resolution esophageal pressure topography (EPT). Am J Gastroenterol. 2012;107(1):37–45.
32. Sperandio M, Tutuian R, Gideon RM, et al. Diffuse esophageal spasm: not diffuse but distal esophageal spasm (DES). Dig Dis Sci. 2003;48:1380.
33. Orlando RC, Bozymski EM. Clinical and manometric effects of nitroglycerin in diffuse esophageal spasm. N Engl J Med. 1973;289:23.
34. Swamy N. Esophageal spasm: clinical and manometric response to nitroglycerine and long acting nitrites. Gastroenterology. 1977;72:23.
35. DiMarino AJ Jr. Characteristics of lower esophageal sphincter function in symptomatic diffuse esophageal spasm. Gastroenterology. 1974;66:1.
36. Campo S, Traube M. Lower esophageal sphincter dysfunction in diffuse esophageal spasm. Am J Gastroenterol. 1989;84:928.
37. Pandolfino JE, Roman S, Carlson D, et al. Distal esophageal spasm in high-resolution esophageal pressure topography: defining clinical phenotypes. Gastroenterology. 2011;141:469.
38. Bredenoord AJ, Fox M, Kahrilas PJ, et al. Chicago classification criteria of esophageal motility disorders defined in high resolution esophageal pressure topography. Neurogastroenterol Motil. 2012;24(Suppl 1):57.
39. Spencer HL, Smith L, Riley SA. A questionnaire study to assess long-term outcome in patients with abnormal esophageal manometry. Dysphagia. 2006;21:149.
40. Clouse RE, Lustman PJ, Eckert TC, et al. Low-dose trazodone for symptomatic patients with esophageal contraction abnormalities. A double-blind, placebo-controlled trial. Gastroenterology. 1987;92(4):1027–36.
41. Cannon RO 3rd, Quyyumi AA, Mincemoyer R, et al. Imipramine in patients with chest pain despite normal coronary angiograms. N Engl J Med. 1994;330:1411.
42. Agrawal A, Tutuian R, Hila A, et al. Successful use of phosphodiesterase type 5 inhibitors to control symptomatic esophageal hypercontractility: a case report. Dig Dis Sci. 2005;50:2059.
43. Miller LS, Pullela SV, Parkman HP, et al. Treatment of chest pain in patients with noncardiac, nonreflux, nonachalasia spastic esophageal motor disorders using botulinum toxin injection into the gastroesophageal junction. Am J Gastroenterol. 2002;97:1640.
44. Minami H, Isomoto H, Yamaguchi N, et al. Peroral esophageal myotomy (POEM) for diffuse esophageal spasm. Endoscopy. 2014;46(S 01):E79–81.
45. Agrawal A, Hila A, Tutuian R, et al. Clinical relevance of the nutcracker esophagus: suggested revision of criteria for diagnosis. J Clin Gastroenterol. 2006;40:504.
46. Korsapati H, Bhargava V, Mittal RK. Reversal of asynchrony between circular and longitudinal muscle contraction in nutcracker esophagus by atropine. Gastroenterology. 2008;135:796.
47. Cattau EL Jr, Castell DO, Johnson DA, et al. Diltiazem therapy for symptoms associated with nutcracker esophagus. Am J Gastroenterol. 1991;86:272.
48. Vanuytsel T, Bisschops R, Farré R, et al. Botulinum toxin reduces dysphagia in patients with nonachalasia primary esophageal motility disorders. Clin Gastroenterol Hepatol. 2013;11:1115.

49. Patti MG, Gorodner MV, Galvani C, et al. Spectrum of esophageal motility disorders: implications for diagnosis and treatment. Arch Surg. 2005;140(5):442–8.
50. Zamost BJ, Hirschberg J, Ippoliti AF, et al. Esophagitis in scleroderma. Prevalence and risk factors. Gastroenterology. 1987;92:421.
51. Yarze JC, Varga J, Stampfl D, et al. Esophageal function in systemic sclerosis: a prospective evaluation of motility and acid reflux in 36 patients. Am J Gastroenterol. 1993;88:870.
52. Poirier NC, Taillefer R, Topart P, et al. Antireflux operations in patients with scleroderma. Ann Thorac Surg. 1994;58(1):66–72.
53. Watson DI, Jamieson GG, Bessell JR, et al. Laparoscopic fundoplication in patients with an aperistaltic esophagus and gastroesophageal reflux. Dis Esophagus. 2006;19(2):94–8.
54. Kent MS, Luketich JD, Irshad K, et al. Comparison of surgical approaches to recalcitrant gastroesophageal reflux disease in the patient with scleroderma. Ann Thorac Surg. 2007;84(5):1710–5.
55. Galmiche JP, Clouse RE, Balint A, Cook IJ, Kahrilas PJ, Paterson WG, et al. Functional esophageal disorders. Gastroenterology. 2006;130(5):1459–65.
56. Herregods TVK, van Hoeji FB, Bredenord AJ, Smout AJPM. Subtle lower esophageal relaxation abdnormalities in patients with unexplained esophageal dysphagia. Neurogastroenterol Motil. 2017;30(2):e13188.
57. Cook IJ, Dent J, Shannon S, Collins SM. Measurement of upper esophageal sphincter pressure. Effect of acute emotional stress. Gastroenterology. 1987;93(3):526–32.
58. Hirano I, Moy N, Heckman MG, Thomas CS, Gonsalves N, Achem SR. Endoscopic assessment of the oesophageal features of eosinophilic oesophagitis: validation of a novel classification and grading system. Gut. 2013;62:489–95.
59. Dellon ES, Gonsalves N, Hirano I, et al. ACG clinical guideline: evidenced based approach to the diagnosis and management of esophageal eosinophilia and eosinophilic esophagitis (EoE). Am J Gastroenterol. 2013;108:679.
60. Prasad GA, Talley NJ, Romero Y, et al. Prevalence and predictive factors of eosinophilic esophagitis in patients presenting with dysphagia: a prospective study. Am J Gastroenterol. 2007;102:2627.
61. McElhiney J, Lohse MR, Arora AS, Peloquin JM, Geno DM, Kuntz MM, Enders FB, et al. The Mayo Dysphagia Questionnaire-30: documentation of reliability and validity of a tool for interventional trials in adults with esophageal disease. Dysphagia. 2010;25:221–30.
62. Straumann A, Conus S, Degen L, et al. Long-term budesonide maintenance treatment is partially effective for patients with eosinophilic esophagitis. Clin Gastroenterol Hepatol. 2011;9:400.
63. Wolf WA, Cotton CC, Green DJ, et al. Predictors of response to steroid therapy for eosinophilic esophagitis and treatment of steroid-refractory patients. Clin Gastroenterol Hepatol. 2015;13:452.

Reoperative Surgery for Failed Antireflux Procedures

3

Kenan Ulualp and Jon C. Gould

Introduction

Gastroesophageal reflux disease (GERD) is a common condition in the Western world with a prevalence of approximately 40% [1]. Nearly 5% of all visits to a primary care provider's office are related to GERD [2]. Some patients develop symptoms or complications of GERD that prove refractory to medical management and choose to undergo antireflux surgery. Laparoscopic Nissen fundoplication is the current gold standard with patient satisfaction reported to be as high as 90% [3]. Published literature suggests that approximately 5–10% of patients eventually undergo reoperative surgery following an antireflux procedure for a variety of indications including persistent, recurrent, or new onset symptoms [4, 5]. Reoperative antireflux surgery can be quite difficult due to adhesions, obscured anatomy, and more advanced disease. Morbidity rates can be high, and satisfaction is decreased with revisions when compared to primary fundoplication [6, 7]. In addition, the likelihood of subsequent revisions increases with each additional attempt at correction [8]. These facts combine to make reoperative antireflux surgery a high stakes intervention. A thorough understanding of the potential mechanisms of failure of the original procedure, the appropriate preoperative evaluation, and the selection of the appropriate reoperative procedure including an intimate knowledge of the techniques for dealing with intraoperative and postoperative challenges is essential to achieving a good outcome.

K. Ulualp, M.D.
Division of Gastroenterology, Medical College of Wisconsin, Milwaukee, WI, USA

J. C. Gould, M.D. (✉)
Division of General Surgery, Medical College of Wisconsin, Milwaukee, WI, USA
e-mail: jgould@mcw.edu

© Springer International Publishing AG, part of Springer Nature 2018
D. Oleynikov, P. M. Fisichella (eds.), *A Mastery Approach to Complex Esophageal Diseases*, https://doi.org/10.1007/978-3-319-75795-7_3

Risk Factors Contributing to Surgical Failure

Failure of an antireflux surgical procedure may be either immediate or delayed and following an interval of relative efficacy that can range from weeks to years. In addition, failure may be related to a persistance or recurrence of the original symptoms that led to the decision to perform an antireflux procedure, or failure may be primarily related to new symptoms (dysphagia as a new symptom following surgery for example). In some cases, symptomatic failure is related to an improper diagnosis or poor operative indication.

In general, patients with a poor response to adequate acid suppression medical therapy, unusual or atypical symptoms, and those with a normal preoperative pH study are more likely to be dissatisfied with the symptomatic outcomes of antireflux surgery [9]. For patients whose symptoms fail to respond to an antireflux procedure, consideration should be given to whether antireflux surgery was indicated and if the preoperative evaluation was complete and appropriate. Eosinophilic esophagitis, achalasia, and functional heartburn are conditions that may seem like GERD that can be missed without a proper preoperative evaluation. Patients with these conditions who undergo antireflux surgery will not be satisfied with the symptomatic outcome and side effects of antireflux surgery. A proper preoperative workup should include a barium swallow, upper endoscopy, esophageal manometry, and a pH study [10].

When the evaluation and indications for antireflux surgery are appropriate, failure can also be the result of technical errors by the surgeon. A fundoplication that is too tight, too long, twisted, constructed with the wrong part of the stomach, or placed in the wrong location below the gastroesophageal junction will not function appropriately and is highly likely to result in dysphagia or other symptoms [11, 12]. Closing the hiatus too tight can result in hiatal stenosis and esophageal outflow obstruction with dysphagia [13]. Creating a geometrically correct fundoplication in the correct location relative to the gastroesophageal junction is a key to good symptomatic outcomes. The internal diameter of the fundoplicaiton should exceed the external diameter of the esophagus as well. This is largely depenant on proper technique in fundoplication construction [14].

Even when constructed appropriately, a fundoplication can fail. Patients who fall into this category of failure often feel well for a period of time before experiencing recurrent or new symptoms. One retrospective analysis of patients with a failed fundoplication revealed that diaphragm stressors such as gagging, retching, and vomiting in the perioperative period represents a major risk factor for anatomic failure with slipped and/or herniated fundoplication [15]. Morbid obesity is also a significant risk factor for anatomic fundoplicaiton failure [16]. For morbidly obese patients, a more appropriate operation for GERD is likely a Roux-en Y gastric bypass rather than a fundoplication [17]. The esophageal hiatus is a 'hostile environment' for a fundoplicaiton. The diaphragm is a thin muscle that is constantly in motion. The hiatal defect cannot be closed or covered, and the pressure differential between the abdomen and the chest is perpetually pushing the fundoplicaiton cephelad. The majority of anatomic failures of previously functional fundoplications are

Table 3.1 Etiology for failure of an antireflux procedure

Misdiagnosis
Achalasia
Eosinophilic esophagitis
Functional heartburn or dyspepsia
Extraesophageal symptom (cough, hoarse voice, etc.) not secondary to GERD
Functional problems
Severe esophageal dysmotility
Gastroparesis
Other esophageal motility disorders such as nutcracker esophagus or diffuse esophageal spasm
Primary technical problems
Fundoplication too tight
Fundoplication twisted
Fundoplication in wrong location relative to gastroesophageal junction
Hiatus closed too tight
Vagal nerve injury and gastroparesis
Anatomic failure
Fundoplication slip
Fundoplication disruption
Herniated fundoplication/hiatal hernia

related to herniation of the intact fundoplication through the hiatus for these reasons [18]. Reasons for failure of an antireflux procedure are listed in Table 3.1.

Clinical Presentation

The clinical presentation of a patient with a failed fundoplication is related to the mechanism of failure as described above. In patients with failed fundoplication due to an incorrect diagnosis, presentation may simply be a persistence of symptoms previously attributed to GERD despite an anatomically intact fundoplication. In some patients with an incorrect diagnosis, the clinical presentation may be persistence or even worsening of the primary symptom(s) and the onset of new symptoms. Missed achalasia is a classic example of the latter. Many patients with achalasia will experience regurgitation and heartburn (intraesophageal reflux and stasis) and initially undergo treatment with acid suppression assuming that the diagnosis is GERD. When acid suppression fails to control the symptoms, these patients may be referred for antireflux surgery. Performing a fundoplication around a non-relaxing lower esophageal sphincter in the setting of aperistalsis leads to even more problems with these issues. This demonstrates the importance of a proper preoperative workup.

In patients whose fundoplication is improperly performed (too tight, twisted, around the stomach rather than the esophagus), symptoms usually persist or may be worse. Many of these patients also describe dysphagia related to impaired esophageal emptying. Some patients suffer from extreme bloating post-fundoplication, which can be a real debilitating problem in some cases. Bloating and difficulty belching is a common complaint following fundoplication, especially in the first 6 months. This may be related to eating too fast, drinking carbonated beverages, lactose intolerance, gastroparesis (existing prior to fundoplication or secondary to vagal nerve injury at the time of fundoplication), irritable bowel, bacterial overgrowth, celiac disease, or a multitude of other issues.

In patients whose fundoplication fails after an interval of good symptom control, anatomic failure is typically the cause and these patients may present with a recurrence of their preoperative symptoms and perhaps with dysphagia if esophageal emptying is impaired by the anatomic failure.

Clinical Evaluation

The evaluation of a patient with a failed fundoplication begins with a thorough assessment of the indications and a review of the preoperative testing conducted prior to the preceding procedure. Upper endoscopy reports, upper GI images, esophageal manometry and pH study reports and in some cases the raw data can be helpful in determining if the original procedure performed was an appropriate choice. This is especially important when the surgeon considering a reoperation for a failed fundoplication did not perform the original procedure. A review of the previous operative report is helpful as well. Details from the operative report that can be useful include comments regarding the size of any hiatal hernia and extent of mediastinal mobilization performed, difficulty encountered closing the hiatus, technique used to close the hiatus, presence of mesh (including what type, configuration, location, fixation method), whether a bougie was used and what size, what kind of fundoplication was performed, and so on can help the reoperative surgeon with orientation and wayfinding during the often difficult disseciton in reoperative cases.

Upper GI Esophogram: We attain an upper GI esophogram and an upper endoscopy in all potential reoperative antireflux surgery patients. An upper GI can help demonstrate the anatomy and evaluate for the presence of a hiatal hernia. A timed barium esophogram with a marshmallow challenge is helpful in patients with dysphagia after a fundoplication to determine if there is a degree of esophageal stasis and impaired emptying that may account for these symptoms. Figure 3.1 is an image from an upper GI series that demonstrates a slipped fundoplicaiton that has herniated above the diaphragm.

Upper Endoscopy: Upper endoscopy prior to reoperative antireflux surgery is essential. An upper endoscopy can identify mucosal changes such as erosive esophagitis, ulcers, Barrett's metaplasia, or other lesions or pathology. Eosinophilic esophagitis and candida esophagitis may be identified and should be treated prior to revisional surgery. The presence of permanent sutures related to the prior fundoplicaiton or mesh at the hiatus in the lumen of the esophagus or stomach should be documented. The location of the hiatus and of the fundoplication should be noted. In patients with esophageal outflow obstruction and stasis, partially

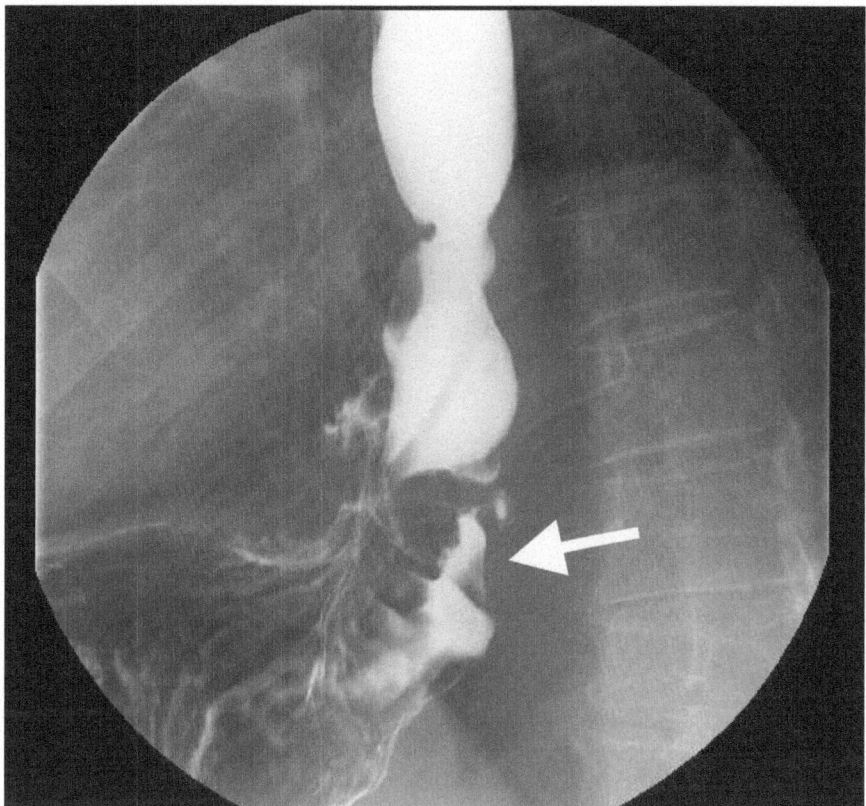

Fig. 3.1 Slipped fundoplication and hiatal hernia

digested food and secretions may be pooled in the esophagus. In patients with vagal nerve injury and post-surgical gastroparesis, a bezoar or partially digested food may be noted in the stomach. The configuraiton of the fundoplication itself should be noted on retroflex view with the endoscope. The mechanism of failure can often be determined with this maneuver that can reveal a paraesophageal hernia or an intrathoracic, twisted, disrupted, or a slipped fundoplication [19]. Figure 3.2 is a retroflex view from an endoscopy that shows a paraesophageal hernia and a fundoplication.

Gastric emptying study: Following truncal vagotomy for peptic ulcer disease, the incidence of post-surgical gastroparesis may be as high as 5% [20]. The exact incidence of postsurgical gastroparesis in patients undergoing laparoscopic fundoplication is much lower than that and hard to define based on the literature. The fact that delayed gastric emptying can be a complication following laparoscopic antireflux surgery is well described based on numerous published case series of patients suffering from post-surgical gastroparesis [21]. In patients with symptoms consistent with gastroparesis (nausea, vomiting, severe bloating, early and prolonged satiety), or in patients with retained food in the stomach on upper endoscopy, a

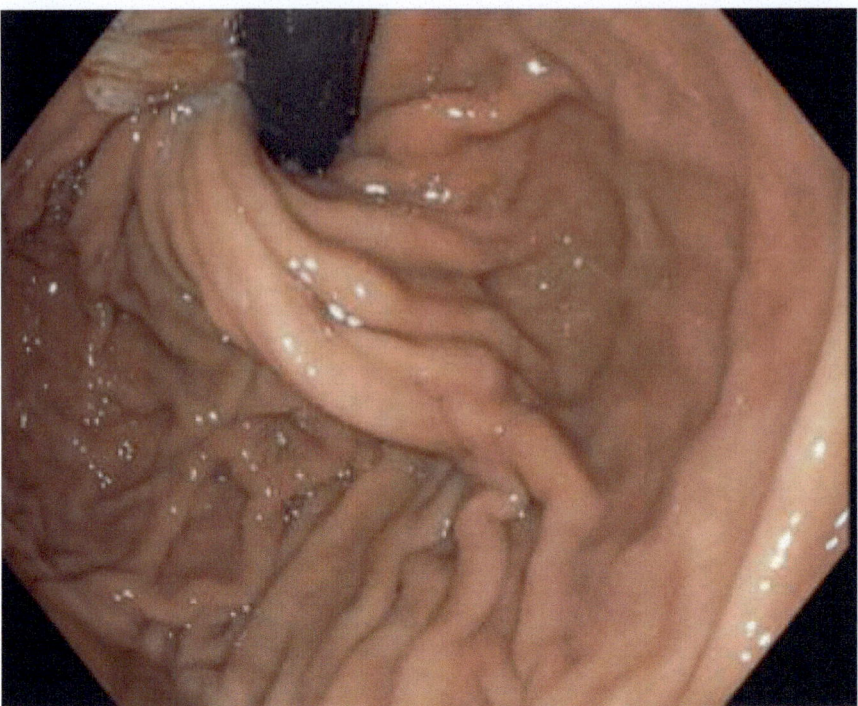

Fig. 3.2 Upper Endoscopy and retroflex view of slipped fundoplication

nuclear medicine gastric emptying study should be attained. In a patient with significant symptoms of gastroparesis and delayed gastric emptying on a nuclear medicine study, consideration should be given to a concurrent pyloroplasty of possibly even a Roux-en Y gastric bypass as a salvage operation (discussed in following sections).

Esophageal manometry: Esophageal manometry is indicated in patients with severe dysphagia and especially in cases where a manometry was not attained prior to the index operation. In general, one should err on the side of performing as thorough a preoperative assessment as possible given the high stakes of reoperative antireflux surgery. In cases where the esophageal motility is ineffective, consideration can be given to a partial fundoplication, such as a Toupet.

Esophageal pH monitoring: Esophageal pH monitoring can help confirm that symptoms following a previous antireflux operation are reflux related. This can be especially helpful in patients with persistent symptoms following antireflux surgery. In patient with unusual symptoms following a prior antireflux procedure, a pH study can provide additional information to support a decision to proceed with reoperative surgery or to pursue alternative diagnosis or treatments.

In general, the evaluation prior to reoperative antireflux surgery is similar to that attained prior to a primary antireflux procedure, with additional tests depending on the nature of the patient's symptoms [22].

Operative Approaches

Reoperative antireflux surgery is a complex procedure and requires a great deal of skill, experience, and judgement to obtain an optimal outcome. We have noted in our large clinical experience that the number of prior reoperative antireflux surgical attempts in a given patient is directly related to the perioperative morbidity and inversely related to the symptomatic and functional outcomes. In these author's opinions, reoperative antireflux surgery is best performed at high volume centers and by surgeons with significant experience in reoperative foregut surgery for these reasons.

Selecting the appropriate procedure based on the patient's medical and surgical history, the mechanism of failure(s) of prior procedure(s), and the results of a thorough preoperative evaluation is critical for success. Rough guidelines we use to decide on the optimal procedure are depicted in Fig. 3.3. In general, morbidly obese patients with a failed fundoplication should ideally undergo takedown of the prior fundoplication, repair of a hiatal hernia if present, and conversion to a Roux-en Y gastric bypass. As noted, obesity is a significant risk factor for fundoplication failure. A reoperative fundoplication in the setting of morbid obesity is likely to fail. A gastric bypass is a highly effective GERD operation [23]. When fundoplications fail anatomically, the incidence of repeat failures may be as high as 20–30% and likely increases with each subsequent attempt at reoperative fundoplication [24, 25]. Little and colleagues reported that although satisfactory results were achieved after initial reoperation in 84% of patients, these satisfactory results declined to 42% in patients who had undergone three or more operations [26]. We believe that when there have been two or more failed fundoplication attempts that consideration should be given to converting to a Roux en Y gastric bypass. In the setting of symptomatic gastroparesis, either a pyloroplasty of a conversion to a gastric bypass should be considered. In patients with symptomatic gastroparesis, Roux en Y gastric bypass has been demonstrated to result in an improvement in gastroparesis-related symptoms [27].

Our preferred approach to these procedures in almost all cases is laparoscopic. There are advantages in terms of decreased wound complications (hernias and infections) and postoperative pain and recovery for a laparoscopic compared to an open approach. With a laparoscope, visualization and mobilization of the stomach and esophagus high into the mediastinum is attainable to a degree not possible with an abdominal laparotomy. Some surgeons prefer the to use the surgical robot for these reoperative cases, but our bias is that the tactile feedback and ability to rapidly and frequently change instruments with standard laparoscopy is an important feature of our preferred approach.

Reoperative fundoplication: Reoperative fundoplication involves taking down the previous fundoplication completely in nearly all patients. Abdominal access for laparoscopy is attained with a Veress needle in the left subcostal area in the midclavicular line. Upon successful insufflation, a 5-mm optical viewing bladeless trocar is used to access the abdomen through the Veress site. A total of four 5-mm ports are used. If mesh at the hiatus is removed or placed, the left subcostal port is upsized to 10-mm. A subxiphoid Nathanson liver retractor is placed in all patients.

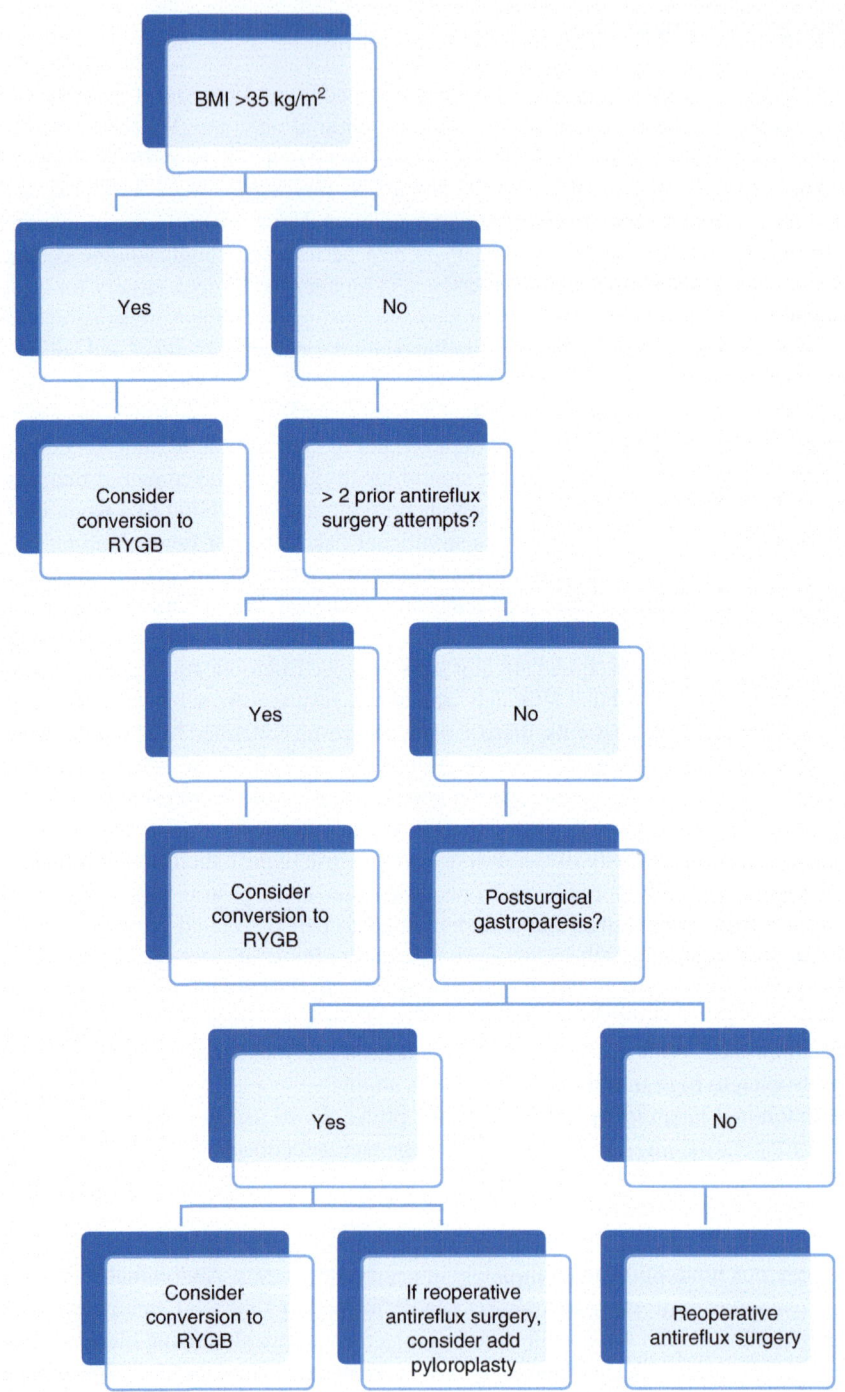

Fig. 3.3 Decision tree for choosing an appropriate procedure after a previous failed antireflux procedure

Adhesiolysis involves a combination of sharp dissection with a scissors, dissection with an ultrasonic shears, and blunt dissection with a laparoscopic suction irrigator tip where appropriate. When technically feasible, the caudate lobe of the liver is identified first, which allows for identification of the right crus of the diaphragm. Dissection typically starts at the base of the right crus and proceeds anteriorly in the plane between the right crus and the fundus/esophagus if possible. Ultimately, the fundoplication or esophagus is circumferentially mobilized off the hiatal muscle—preserving as much muscle and fascia as possible on the diaphragm. In some cases with severe and dense adhesions, the anatomic landmark that proves easiest to find is the base of the left crus and this is after dividing branches or the gastroepiploic vessels to the body of the stomach and entering the lesser sac posterior to the stomach and somewhat removed from the operative site and hiatal adhesions.

In cases with pre-existing mesh at the hiatus, the mesh is removed in its entirety when possible. Care is taken to preserve as much diaphragm muscle as possible when removing mesh. Care is also taken to ensure that mesh adherent to the fundus or esophagus can be safely removed without damage or perforation to the foregut. Mesh excision from the esophagus or fundus is almost always done sharply with scissors. Sometimes, more than one fresh scissors tip is needed in these cases. A sharp scissors tip is essential.

Once the fundus or esophagus is freed from the hiatus, the fundoplication is taken down. Usually, the fundoplication sutures can be visualized and a combination of dissection with an ultrasonic energy source or with scissors is utilized to dismantle the fundoplication. Ultrasonic shears are only used when the sutures and tissue planes can be clearly visualized. An advantage to using the shears in this context is better hemostasis but also a 'cavitation' effect that can facilitate the dissection and help to identify tissue planes. A disadvantage to the ultrasonic shears is the fact that tissue injury and perhaps delayed perforation is a potential consequence. Fundus to fundus, fundus to esophagus, and ultimately fundus to retroperitoneum/diaphragm adhesions are carefully taken down until the greater curve of the stomach and angle of His is restored to its native anatomic position.

Circumferential and high mediastinal mobilization of the esophagus is performed until 2–4 cm of intra-abdominal esophageal length can be attained without tension. A Penrose drain around the esophagus is used for gentle retraction. The vagus nerves are identified and preserved when possible. Esophageal lengthening procedures are rarely necessary. When needed, we perform a laparoscopic wedge fundectomy for a Collis gastroplasty as described by others [28].

Primary crural repairs are performed in all patients. In patients with a dilated hiatus or loss of muscle at the hiatus from the dissection, a right-sided crural relaxing incision is performed to allow for primary closure. To perform a relaxing incision, a hook cautery or ultrasonic shears is used to incise the right crus of the diaphragm starting about 2–3 mm medial to the vena cava when possible. A full thickness muscle incision is made and if possible the right pleural cavity is not entered. In most cases good medialization of the right crura is possible without opening the pleura. In cases where the pleura is entered, the pleura on the right side is opened through the hiatus and a 19Fr silastic drain is placed through the hiatus anteriorly, into the mediastinum, and into the right chest. At the end of the case, this drain is externalized through a 5-mm port. The anesthesiologist then gives several big Valsalva breaths with the ventilator as the drain is slowly removed under suction. Chest tubes or abdominal drains are not routinely left in place in these cases.

In patients undergoing reoperative fundoplication in whom the hiatal repair is determined to be under tension or for whom a crural relaxing incision is needed, a U-shaped piece of synthetic bioabsorbable mesh (Gore Bio-A, Flagstaff, AZ) is used to reinforce the hiatal repair and sutured into place. In patients with pre-existing dysphagia or impaired esophageal motility (based on manometry), a posterior partial fundoplication (Toupet) is constructed. In patients to undergo reconstruction of a Nissen fundoplication, a 56–60 French esophageal bougie is utilized. Gastropexy sutures between the fundoplication, the posterior hiatal repair, and the anterior left and right crural pillars are routinely placed. Endoscopy is performed liberally during the procedure to help identify the anatomy and to ensure there are no unrecognized perforations. Endoscopy is performed at the end of the procedure to ensure the same and that the fundoplication is in the right location relative to the gastroesophageal junction and that the geometry of the wrap on retroflexion is appropriate.

Conversion to Roux-en Y gastric Bypass: In patients undergoing conversion to gastric bypass, much of the initial procedure is as described above for the reoperative fundoplication. There are a total of five ports, with two of them being 10-mm to accommodate the linear cutting stapler. The previous fundoplication is always taken down and any hiatal mesh is removed as described.

The gastric pouch is created from the proximal stomach and is approximately 30 mL. The lesser curve neurovascular bundle is preserved. The left gastric artery is always identified and the pouch is created below this artery to ensure an adequate blood supply. In select cases with multiple previous fundoplication attempts undergoing conversion to gastric bypass, indocyanine green (ICG) is administered intravenously to help identify the left gastric artery and branches, and to ensure that the proposed pouch has adequate perfusion prior to firing the laparoscopic stapler. A laparoscopic camera system with near infrared imaging capabilities (Stryker 1588 Advanced Imaging Modalities Platform, Stryker, Kalamazoo, MI/USA) is used for this purpose. Resection of a portion of proximal fundus is undertaken if intraoperative perforation occurs, or if the blood supply to this portion of the fundus is questionable following creation of the proximal gastric pouch. New mesh at the hiatus is avoided in these reoperative cases undergoing conversion to gastric bypass.

A 50-cm biliopancreatic limb, antecolic and antegastric 100-cm Roux limb (150-cm for those with a BMI > 50), and a linear stapled gastrojejunostomy are constructed. The gastrojejunostomy is completed with a 32-Fr bougie in place and the entire stapled anastomosis is over-sewn with absorbable Vicryl sutures. The gastric pouch is sutured to the hiatal closure posteriorly and to the anterior left and right crural pillar as described for the reoperative fundoplication procedures. As in the reoperative fundoplication procedures, endoscopy is performed liberally and often to help guide the creation of the pouch, to identify the anatomy, and to ensure the gastrojejunostomy is hemostatic, without leak, and easy to traverse with an endoscope.

Outcomes

When the best procedure is performed well and for the proper indications, outcomes of reoperative antireflux surgery are excellent. A recently published comprehensive review of reoperative fundoplications revealed that in 17 included studies involving more than 1000 patients, that the most common indication for reoperative fundoplication was recurrent GERD (59%), most often secondary to fundoplication herniation [29]. The second most common indication for reoperative surgery was dysphagia (31%). Intra-operative complications occurred in 18.6% of cases and were most commonly gastrointestinal perforations. Success rates, defined variably, were 81%. The authors of another systematic review included 81 studies and more than 4500 patients and reached similar conclusions, but also felt that morbidity and mortality after redo surgery was higher than after primary surgery and symptomatic and objective outcome were less satisfactory [18].

In certain circumstances, Roux en Y gastric bypass has been demonstrated to be the best salvage procedure after failed fundoplication, even in patients who are not obese. Morbid obesity, poor esophageal motility, delayed gastric emptying, and multiple previous surgeries at the hiatus have been proposed as risk factors for a poor clinical outcome with reoperative fundoplication after failed fundoplication. Yamamato et al. retrospectively reviewed their experience of 119 reoperative fundoplications and 64 RYGB after a previous failed fundoplication attempt [25]. Patients with the aforementioned risk factors underwent gastric bypass rather than an attempt at fundoplication. Despite the fact that patients undergoing gastric bypass had a significantly higher body mass index, higher number of risk factors, and higher preoperative severity of heartburn and regurgitation compared to the reoperative fundoplication group, symptom severity improved to a similar degree following both procedures.

Failure of Reoperative Fundoplication

As described previously, when reoperative fundoplications fail, the incidence of repeated failures escalates. The morbidity increases with each additional attempt at repair and the chance of an optimal symptomatic outcome gradually declines. Some patients with failed reoperative procedures may be better off with persistent or recurrent symptoms managed medically to whatever degree is possible as opposed to yet another attempt at surgical correction. Risk factors that may be contributing to multiple failures should be addressed when possible before proceeding with yet another attempt. Smoking cessation and preoperative weight loss are two of the more common modifiable risk factors. Proper procedure selection is critical. Only surgeons and teams with a large experience and focused expertise in reoperative antireflux surgery should attempt reoperative surgery for a previously failed fundoplication. In patients with three or more failed prior antireflux procedures that require surgery, the salvage procedure of choice is almost always a conversion to a gastric bypass. In these patients we spend a great deal of time discussing the risks and options and setting realistic goals for symptomatic outcomes. We also discuss the possibility that salvage of a vascularized proximal gastric pouch may not be possible and an esophagojejunostomy may occasionally be necessary. When we are forced to perform an esophagojejunostomy, we place a feeding jejunostomy tube during the procedure. In nearly all patients, we are able to advance their diet and gradually wean tube feedings to the point where the jejunostomy tube can be removed by approximately 3 months postoperatively.

Conclusions

Reoperative antireflux surgery is a complex and high stakes intervention best done well the first time. Indications for reoperative surgery include fundoplication failure due to incorrect preoperative diagnosis, improper technique or choice of primary procedure, and delayed anatomic failure. A proper evaluation prior to reoperative surgery is critical for operative decision-making and a good outcome.

References

1. Ronkainen J, Aro P, Storskrubb T, et al. High prevalence of gastroesophageal reflux symptoms and esophagitis with or without symptoms in the general adult Swedish population: a Kalixanda study report. Scand J Gastroenterol. 2005;40(3):275–85.
2. Liker H, Hungin P, Wiklund I. Managing gastroesophageal reflux disease in primary care: the patient perspective. J Am Board Fam Pract. 2005;18(5):393–400.
3. Gee DW, Andreoli MT, Rattner DW. Measuring the effectiveness of laparoscopic antireflux surgery: long-term results. Arch Surg. 2008;143(5):482–7.
4. Funch-Jensen P, Bendixen A, Gerding Iversen M, Jensen HK. Complications and frequency of redo antireflux surgery in Denmark: a nationwide study, 1997-2005. Surg Endosc. 2008;22:627–30.
5. Hatch KF, Daily MF, Christensen BJ, Glasgow RE. Failed fundoplications. Am J Surg. 2004;188(6):786–91.
6. Musunuru S, Gould JC. Perioperative outcomes of surgical procedures for symptomatic fundoplication failure: a retrospective case-control study. Surg Endosc. 2012;26(3):838–42.
7. DePaula AL, Hashiba K, Bafutto M, Machado CA. Laparoscopic reoperations after failed and complicated antireflux operations. Surg Endosc. 1995;9:681–6.
8. Smith CD, McClusky DA, Abu Rajad M, Lederman AB, Hunter JG. When fundoplication fails: redo? Ann Surg. 2005;241(6):861–9.
9. Davis CS, Baldea A, Johns JR, Joehl RJ, Fisichella PM. The evolution and long-term results of laparoscopic antireflux surgery for the treatment of gastroesophageal reflux disease. JSLS. 2010;14(3):332–41.
10. Jobe BA, Richter JE, Hoppo T, et al. Preoperative diagnostic workup before antireflux surgery: an evidence and experience-based consensus of the Esophageal Diagnostic Advisory Panel. J Am Coll Surg. 2013;217(4):586–97.
11. Hunter JG, Smith CD, Branum GD, et al. Laparoscopic fundoplication failures: patterns of failure and response to fundoplication revision. Ann Surg. 1999;230(4):595–604.
12. DeMeester TR, Bonavina L, Albertucci M. Nissen fundoplication for gastroesophageal reflux disease: evaluation of primary repair in 100 consecutive patients. Ann Surg. 1986;204(1):9–20.
13. Granderath FA, Schweiger UM, Kamolz T, Pointner R. Dysphagia after laparoscopic antireflux surgery: a problem of hiatal closure more than a problem of the wrap. Surg Endosc. 2005;19:1439–46.

14. Reardon PR, Matthews BD, Scarborough TK, Preciado A, Marti JL, Kamelgard JI. Geometry and reproducibility in 360 degrees fundoplication. Surg Endosc. 2000;14(8):750–4.
15. Iqbal A, Kakarlapudi GV, Awad ZT, Haynatzki G, Turaga KK, Karu A, Fritz K, Haider M, Mittal SK, Filipi CJ. Assessment of diaphragmatic stressors as risk factors for symptomatic failure of laparoscopic Nissen fundoplication. J Gastrointest Surg. 2006;10(1):12–21.
16. Perez AR, Moncure AC, Rattner DW. Obesity adversely affects the outcome of antireflux operations. Surg Endosc. 2001;15:986–9.
17. Pagé MP, Kastenmeier A, Goldblatt M, Frelich M, Bosler M, Wallace J, Gould J. Medically refractory gastroesophageal reflux disease in the obese: what is the best surgical approach? Surg Endosc. 2014;28(5):1500–4.
18. Van Beek DB, Auyang ED, Soper NJ. A comprehensive review of laparoscopic redo fundoplication. Surg Endosc. 2011;25:706–12.
19. Mittal SK, Juhasz A, Ramanan B, Hoshino M, Lee TH, Filipi CJ. A proposed classification for uniform endoscopic description of surgical fundoplication. Surg Endosc. 2014;28:1103–9.
20. Hasler WL. Gastroparesis: symptoms, evaluation, and treatment. Gastroenterol Clin N Am. 2007;36(3):619–47.
21. Clark CJ, Sarr MG, Arora AS, Nichols FC, Reid-Lombardo KM. Does gastric resection have a role in the management of severe post-fundoplication gastric dysfunction? World J Surg. 2011;35(9):2045–50.
22. Stefanidis D, Hope WW, Kohn GP, Reardon PR, Richardson WS, Fanelli RD, SAGES Guidelines Committee. Guidelines for surgical treatment of gastroesophageal reflux disease. Surg Endosc. 2010;24(11):2647–69.
23. Madalosso CA, Gurski RR, Callegari-Jacques SM, Navarini D, Mazzini G, Pereira Mda S. The impact of gastric bypass on gastroesophageal reflux disease in morbidly obese patients. Ann Surg. 2016;263(1):110–6.
24. Iqbal A, Awad Z, Simkins J, et al. Repair of 104 failed anti-reflux operations. Ann Surg. 2006;244:42–51.
25. Yamamoto SR, Hoshino M, Nandipati KC, Lee TH, Mittal SK. Long-term outcomes of reintervention for failed fundoplication: redo fundoplication versus roux-en-Y reconstruction. Surg Endosc. 2014;28(1):42–8.
26. Little AG, Ferguson MK, Skinner DB. Reoperation for failed antireflux operations. J Thorac Cardiovasc Surg. 1986;91(4):511–7.
27. Papasavas PK, Ng JS, Stone AM, Ajayi OA, Muddasani KP, Tishler DS. Gastric bypass surgery as treatment of recalcitrant gastroparesis. Surg Obes Relat Dis. 2014;10(5):795–9.
28. Zehetner J, DeMeester SR, Ayazi S, Kilday P, Alicuben ET, DeMeester TR. Laparoscopic wedge fundectomy for collis gastroplasty creation in patients with a foreshortened esophagus. Ann Surg. 2014;260(6):1030–3.
29. Furnée EJB, Draaisma WA, Broeders I, Gooszen HG. Surgical reintervention after failed antireflux surgery: a systematic review of the literature. J Gastrointest Surg. 2009;13:1539–49.

Hiatal Hernia and Reflux Following Bariatric Surgery

4

Dietric L. Hennings, Patrick J. McLaren, Samer G. Mattar, and Dmitry Oleynikov

Introduction

Obesity in the United States is rising at alarming rates. More than one out of every three adults in the United States are now classified as obese [1]. Along with this rise in obesity, and with the advent and adoption of laparoscopic principles, the field of bariatric surgery has rapidly expanded in recent years. From 1994 to 2004 the annual number of gastric bypass operations performed in the United States increased 20-fold [2]. In addition to laparoscopic Roux-en-Y gastric bypass (LRYGB), which has been the cornerstone of weight loss surgery for nearly two decades, newer operations are being performed with promising outcomes. Laparoscopic Adjustable Gastric Banding (LAGB) enjoyed popularity through the beginning of the 2000's, but has been almost entirely supplanted in recent years by the Laparoscopic Sleeve Gastrectomy (LSG, Fig. 4.1, Table 4.1) [3]. LSG was initially introduced as a staged operation in patients undergoing a biliopancreatic diversion with duodenal switch operation, but eventually became a stand-alone bariatric procedure. Initial analysis demonstrated LSG had

D. L. Hennings
Department of Surgery, University of Nebraska Medical Center, 986245 Nebraska Medical Center, Omaha, NE, USA

P. J. McLaren
Department of General Surgery, Oregon Health and Science University, Portland, OR, USA

S. G. Mattar
Department of General Surgery, Swedish Medical Center, Seattle, WA, USA
e-mail: Sumeer.Mattar@swedish.org; mattar@ohsu.edu

D. Oleynikov, M.D., F.A.C.S. (✉)

Department of Surgery, University of Nebraska Medical Center, 986245 Nebraska Medical Center, Omaha, NE, USA

Center for Advanced Surgical Technology, University of Nebraska Medical Center, 986245 Nebraska Medical Center, Omaha, NE, USA
e-mail: doleynik@unmc.edu

© Springer International Publishing AG, part of Springer Nature 2018
D. Oleynikov, P. M. Fisichella (eds.), *A Mastery Approach to Complex Esophageal Diseases*, https://doi.org/10.1007/978-3-319-75795-7_4

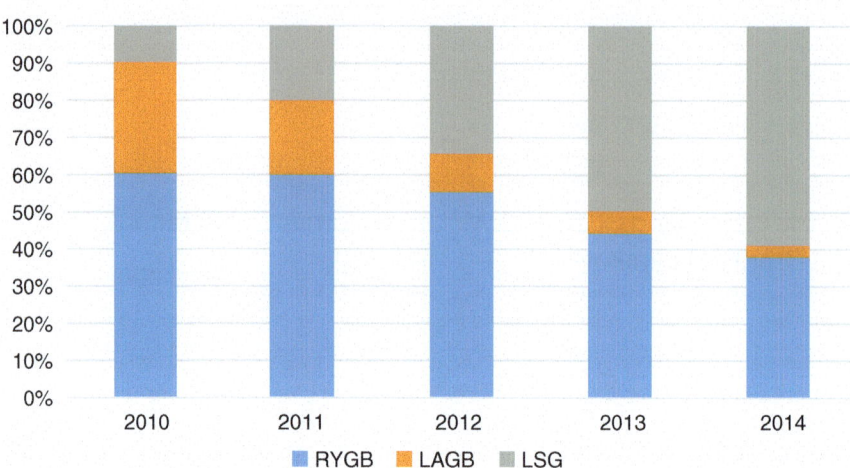

Fig. 4.1 Trends in utilization of different surgical approaches to bariatric surgery in the United States, 2010–2014. Data from the American College of Surgeons National Surgical Quality Improvement Program database. Image adapted from [3]. RYGB, Roux-en-Y Gastric Bypass; LAGB, laparoscopic gastric band; LSG, laparoscopic sleeve gastrectomy

improved weight loss and metabolic outcomes compared to LAGB, even approaching those of LRYGB [4]. Long-term data is still being evaluated to determine the durability of LSG. Due to a lower complication and reoperation rate and the relative simplicity of the procedure compared to gastric bypass, LSG now accounts for the largest proportion of bariatric operations performed in the U.S. and worldwide [3, 4]. Surgical weight loss procedures are not equivalent, each having its own morbidity and mortality profile and perioperative management strategies. For the bariatric patient with gastroesophageal reflux disease (GERD), LRYGB can improve symptoms in the vast majority of patients [5]. LSG on the other hand, while improving pre-existing GERD in some patients, can cause (*de novo* GERD) or aggravate pre-existing reflux. Inadequate weight loss and uncontrolled GERD are the most common indications for revisional bariatric surgery. Additionally, hiatal hernias occur in up to 50% of patients after LSG and are a significant contributor to post-operative reflux [6]. In this chapter, we will discuss the assessment and management options for patients with GERD and hiatal hernia in the setting of bariatric surgery.

Table 4.1 Emerging prevalence of SG in diminishing LRYGB

	2011	2012	2013	2014	2015	2016
Total	158,000	173,000	179,000	193,000	196,000	216,000
LRYGB	36.7%	37.5%	34.2%	26.8%	23.1%	18.7%
Band	35.4%	20.2%	14%	9.5%	5.7%	3.4%
Sleeve	17.8%	33%	42.1%	51.7%	53.8%	58.1%
BPD/DS	0.9%	1%	1%	0.4%	0.6%	0.6%
Revisions	6%	6%	6%	11.5%	13.6%	9.7%
Other	3.2%	2.3%	2.7%	0.1%	3.2%	6.9%
Balloons					~700 cases	2.7%
V-Bloc					18 cases	

Preoperative Assessment

The most important aspect of minimizing complications following bariatric surgery is identifying and mitigating patient risk factors pre-operatively. In addition to bariatric-specific considerations, patients considering weight loss surgery should be assessed following a standardized and comprehensive protocol. Patient selection should be based on a multidisciplinary team approach, evaluating patient comorbidities, nutritional education, a psychological evaluation for coping mechanisms and pathologic eating habits, and evaluation for surgical fitness. Often, patients have conducted their own research of bariatric procedures and express a preference. The surgeon must adequately inform the patient on expected outcomes of each potential procedure and any potential complications and reach a shared decision with the patient on the appropriateness of a particular surgical option [7]. Medical comorbidities should be fully investigated including possible cardiac work up, evaluation for reflux disease or hiatal hernia, and special considerations such as underlying kidney or liver disease.

GERD is present in up to 61% of the bariatric population [8]. The bariatric preoperative assessment should include a thorough history and physical exam with direct questioning regarding GERD symptoms and history of antacid medication use. Further evaluation should be considered for patients on antisecretory medications (PPI, H2 blockers), a history of peptic or duodenal ulcer, history of *H. pylori* infection, or severe symptoms of reflux. Investigational studies usually consist of an EGD with or without biopsy, manometry, upper GI series, or 24-hour pH monitoring. While no definitive consensus exists on the role of manometry and pH monitoring prior to bariatric surgery, such studies can help delineate esophageal pathology that may be mistaken for GERD symptoms. There appears to be significant correlation between BMI, waist circumference and axial separation of the lower esophageal sphincter (LES) and crura, resulting in decreased LES pressure, impaired esophageal clearance and increased sensitivity to transient lower esophageal sphincter relaxation (TLESR) [9, 10]. Upper endoscopy is a valuable tool to rule out gastritis, ulceration, Barrett's esophagus, dysplasia, and malignant lesions. Abnormal findings on endoscopy that change the surgical approach or delay the operation have been shown to occur in 12–60% of patients [11]. Since LRYGB excludes much of the stomach and all of the duodenum, post-operative endoscopic surveillance of the distal stomach and duodenum is significantly more complicated, and best performed prior to surgery.

The presence of a hiatal hernia is another valuable finding that can be identified on endoscopy which may alter the surgical approach. Hiatus hernia requiring concurrent repair has been shown to be present in 5–50% of patients undergoing pre-operative endoscopy for bariatric surgery [12]. The bariatric patient is at increased risk for hiatal hernia due to increased intra-abdominal pressure causing a trans-diaphragmatic pressure gradient at the gastroesophageal junction (GEJ) weakening the crura and widening the hiatus [13]. Sliding hiatal hernias account for 95% of hiatal hernias and are most commonly associated with GERD [14]. The best (most sensitive? Most specific?) diagnostic study for diagnosis is an upper GI barium study which should be included in the work up of GERD in select bariatric patients.

Reflux Following Adjustable Gastric Band

There are numerous reasons laparoscopic adjustable gastric banding (LAGB) has fallen out of favor. Factors contributing to the decline in LAGB include patient and physician dissatisfaction with the need for frequent maintenance and adjustment visits, modest weight loss profiles, and a high incidence of long-term complications resulting in the requirement for additional surgical procedures and/or device removal.

LAGB-related complications include prolapse or slippage, erosion, port or tubing complications, over-filling of the band causing dysphagia and GERD, esophageal dilation, and weight loss failure. GERD is often present in conjunction with other LAGB-related complications. Diagnostic modalities to rule out band malposition should always be central to evaluation of symptoms after LAGB placement. A plain radiograph will usually show the band in an abnormally horizontal position. Barium swallow will show a significantly greater amount of stomach above the band than would be expected, confirming the prolapse.

LAGB is associated with esophageal motor dysfunction and esophageal dilation, which is perhaps one of the most severe complications that may result from an over-tight or mal-positioned gastric band. Reflux, dysphagia, pain, and food intolerance may be presenting symptoms. Treatment is to remove all fluid from the band, minimizing the restriction and obstruction. Research has shown even with proper placement, esophageal motor dysfunction and dilation persist. Thus, patients may develop refractory symptoms due to non-acid reflux after LAGB [15].

Often the treatment for reflux and other morbidities after LAGB is temporary deflation of the band followed by elective surgical removal of the band, especially when it is the pseudocapsule, ratherthan the band itself, that is contributing to obstructive symptoms. Gastric band repositioning can be an option and should be evaluated in addition to alternative bariatric surgery interventions. Due to conflicting results of studies evaluating LAGB and GERD, many surgeons do not recommend LAGB in a patient with preoperative reflux disease.

Reflux Following Roux-en-Y Gastric Bypass

Roux-en-Y gastric bypass (RYGB) is widely considered the "ideal' anti-reflux procedure, especially in patients with a high BMI, and several studies have reported positive outcomes with GERD, including symptom improvement and reduction in the use of anti-secretory medications [5, 16–18]. Factors improving GERD after RYGB include weight loss, rapid gastric pouch emptying, reduction of parietal cell mass, decreased pressure across the lower esophageal sphincter (LES), and diversion of bilio-pancreatic and gastric secretions. RYGB is superior to all other procedures in improving GERD according to multiple studies [16, 17]. Despite these dramatic results, approximately 20% of patients may have persistent GERD or develop *de novo* reflux [19, 20]. These patients should initially be treated with anti-secretory medications including PPI. If symptoms persist or progress, an EGD may identify additional pathology such as marginal ulceration (most commonly associated with smoking recidivism), esophagitis, gastritis/pouchitis, anatomic stricture or outlet obstruction, large gastric pouch size, or gastrogastric fistula (GGF). If additional pathology is identified, further surgical intervention such as gastrojejunal anastomotic revision, gastric pouch revision, anastomotic dilation, or gastrogastric fistula resection can then be planned. Other proposed mechanisms may be related to ineffective peristaltic waves in the Roux limb due to motor abnormalities of the Roux limb, such as inversion of slow-wave frequency gradient, retrograde slow-wave propagation, or the increased occurrence of ectopic migrating motor complexes [21]. Small bowel follow-through studies will help diagnose inadequate motility. Promotility agents such as metoclopramide, bethanechol, domperidone, and cisapride should be utilized when appropriate.

Prior to anti-reflux intervention, a complete GERD work up including EGD, upper GI barium study, manometry, and 24-hour pH monitoring should be completed. Due to the altered anatomy after RYGB, several endoscopic therapeutic options are available with limited evidence, varying degrees of success and durability. Endoscopic techniques include the LINX® Reflux Management System for magnetic augmentation of the LES (Torax® Medical Inc.; Shoreview, MN USA), radio-frequency energy delivery to the LES (Stretta®; Mederi Therapeutics Inc., Norwalk, CT USA), and electrical stimulation of the LES (EndoStim®; EndoStim Inc., Dallas, TX USA) are under further investigation [22].

GGF remains an important cause of refractory GERD, epigastric pain, and hematemesis in the RYGB patient. This lesion was more common in the era of undivided gastric bypass (usually due to a ruptured staple line). Its incidence has markedly diminished with the adoption of the divided gastric bypass. In the modern era, GGF usually occurs due to a non-healing marginal or gastric ulcer that has penetrated into the excluded stomach. It is more common in patients with a smoking history or those who are predisposed to ulcer formation due to the ingestion of non-steroidal anti-inflammatory agents. The incidence of GGF is 1.5–6% [23–25]. Patients with GGF may present with non-specific symptoms including vomiting, pain and hematemesis. They will also often complain of heartburn, regurgitation (especially when recumbent), halitosis and occasional aspiration episodes. Less common presentation will be weight regain if the fistula enlarges enough to allow the food conduit to preferentially channel through the fistula. Upper GI contrast studies and/or CT scan with oral contrast confirmed the diagnosis in most cases, whereas endoscopy can be falsely negative in a certain number of cases. Initial treatment of GGF can be attempted with proton pump inhibitors, but most symptomatic lesions will require surgical resection, either in isolation, or if the GGF is in proximity to the gastrojejunostomy, with a resection/revision of the gastrojejunostomy. Smaller GGF lesions may be repaired endoscopically with the use of the Overstitch device [26] or certain clips or clamps.

Single-anastomosis gastric bypass, which is also named "mini-gastric bypass" and "omega loop gastric bypass" (OLGB), was originally conceived by Rutledge and has been gaining popularity, especially outside the United States [27]. One of the barriers to its wider adoption in the US has been the concern of bile reflux, which may develop after this operation. Patients with bile reflux present with dyspepsia, esophagitis, anastomotic ulcer or stricture formation. Additionally, there is the serious concern that exposed esophageal epithelium may undergo metaplasia or dysplasia as precursors of esophageal adenocarcinoma. The treatment of choice in these situations has been, in the case of OLGB, to undergo conversion to RYGB [27]. In cases of bile reflux after RYGB, the fact that the Roux limb may be fore-shortened should be contemplated and confirmed with either endoscopy or upper GI contrast radiography. Once diagnosed, patient relief of biliary symptoms can be achieved by translocation of the biliopancreatic limb further downstream along the common alimentary channel.

Reflux Following Sleeve Gastrectomy

Since its introduction, LSG has quickly gained popularity amongst surgeons due its high safety profile and short operative time. Additionally, the operation delivers excellent weight loss outcomes. Resolution of obesity related comorbidities is promising, however the operation has not been widely used in practice for long enough to determine the exact long-term outcomes or complications. A 2017 review of studies with more than 12 months follow up identified 18 studies comparing GERD symptoms before and after LSG [21]. Of those studies, five demonstrated improvement, three showed no change, and ten studies demonstrated worsening of GERD symptoms after LSG. The International Sleeve Gastrectomy Expert Panel reported postoperative GERD symptoms in up to 31% of patients after LSG, with a range in the literature between 2.1 and 34.9% [28]. Similarly, *de novo* GERD following LSG has also been shown to be highly variable ranging from 0 to 45% [28]. Rebecchi et al. conducted the only study to use pH monitoring to objectively measure acid exposure prior to and following LSG. This study demonstrated a significant improvement in both Demeester score and %pH < 4 in patients who had pathologic reflux before surgery [29]. However, the same study noted a 5.4% increase in *de novo* pathologic esophageal acid exposure in patients without GERD before LSG.

It is evident that the development of postoperative GERD is likely multifactorial, but most agree that surgical technique plays a significant role in the prevalence of post-operative GERD [30, 31]. Table 4.2 lists a number of physiologic and anatomical factors that may contribute to the development of GERD after LSG. The LSG procedure is essentially a longitudinal resection of the stomach along the lesser curvature. It is an operation that is relatively simple in concept, but intricate in technique. A variety of subtle maneuvers must be proficiently completed, in order to avoid a lifelong series of complications and misery to the patient. A consensus statement on best practices for surgical technique was proposed by the International Sleeve Gastrectomy Expert Panel in 2011 [28]. These guidelines are summarized in Table 4.3. Two specific technical aspects proposed to reduce post-operative GERD are avoidance of mid-stomach stenosis and careful dissection and division of the stomach at gastroesophageal junction to avoid disruption of the angle of His [29].

Table 4.2 Proposed anatomic and physiologic factors affecting GERD following LSG

Proposed anatomic and physiologic factors affecting GERD following LSG
Worsening GERD
Decreased gastric emptying
Lower LES pressure
Decreased gastric compliance and volume
Increased gastric pressure
Resection of the sling fibers of Helvetius
Blunting angle of his
Stenosis of the gastric outlet
Mid gastric stenosis with proximal distension
Increased gastric pressure
Improving GERD
Accelerated gastric emptying
Weight loss
Restoration of the angle of his
Reduced acid production due to resection of parietal cells
Removal of fundus (source of relaxation waves to lower esophageal sphincter)
Reduced wall tension
Adapted from [32]

Table 4.3 Consensus guidelines on surgical technique when performing LSG from the International Sleeve Gastrectomy Expert Panel. Coral Gables, FL 2011

Consensus guidelines for surgical technique when performing LSG	
Sleeve sizing	Optimal Bougie size is 32–36 French
	Invagination of the staple line reduces lumen size
Stapling	It is not appropriate to use staples with a closed height less than 1.5 mm on any part of sleeve gastrectomy
	When using buttressing materials, surgeons should never use any staple with a closed height less than 2.0 mm
	When resecting the antrum, surgeons should never use any staple with closed height less than 2.0 mm
	Transection should begin 2–6 cm from the pylorus
	It is important to stay away from the GE junction with the last staple firing
Mobilization	It is important to completely mobilize the fundus before transection
Reinforcement	Staple line reinforcement will reduce bleeding along the staple line

Adapted from [28]

Hiatal Hernia and Reflux

Hiatal hernia is a condition that warrants specific consideration for the bariatric surgeon. Symptomatic hiatal hernia is present in 15% of patients with a BMI greater than 35 [33]. The decision to repair a hiatal hernia at the time of bariatric surgery is a subject of some debate. Comparing LSG with hiatal hernia repair versus without repair, most studies fail to show a significant difference in the degree of GERD symptoms post-operatively [34]. While the evidence is mixed on the topic, most surgeons would recommend concomitant repair of moderate to large hiatal hernias at the time of bariatric surgery. If left un-repaired, symptomatic hiatal hernias may obscure more concerning post-operative conditions like staple line leak, ulceration, bowel obstruction, and internal or incisional hernias. Particularly in the post-LSG patient, post-operative hiatal hernias can pose a clinical dilemma. For this reason, it is recommended that repair be undertaken at the time of bariatric surgery.

Interventions for Reflux After Sleeve Gastrectomy

The initial treatment for GERD symptoms following bariatric surgery should be medical. Proton pump inhibitors (PPIs) are effective in controlling symptoms in the majority of patients. However, GERD symptoms that are not controlled with PPIs pose a particular challenge in the LSG patient. Due to the altered anatomy of the GI tract following bariatric surgery, traditional surgical options like fundoplication are not an option. The most effective and durable method for treating GERD in this population is conversion to a LRYGB. Additional treatment options still lack long-term data, although preliminary studies indicate they are likely safe in the bariatric population. These potential treatments include radio-frequency ablation (Stretta, Mederi Therapeutics, Greenwich, CT, United States), magnetic augmentation of LES (LINX® Reflux Management System, Torax Medical, Inc., Shoreview, MN, USA), electrical stimulation therapy of the LES (EndoStim) among other developing technologies.

The most studied and effective option for intractable reflux follow LSG is conversion to RYGB. The general consensus among experts is that RYGB is the best surgical option for bariatric patients with GERD, preoperatively or as a revisional option after other baritric procedures. For patients undergoing revision RYGB for persistent GERD following LSG, symptomatic improvement has been reported in 96–100% of patients [35, 36]. Additionally, avoiding LSG in patients with severe pre-operative GERD has been shown to reduce the need for future revision and conversion to RYGB. As in most cases, revision bariatric surgery is associated with higher morbidity and mortality compared to initial surgery. In experienced hands, revisional cases have acceptable complication profiles.

Conclusion

Bariatric surgery has delivered truly astonishing results for treating metabolic dysfunction and the associated comorbidities. Operation choice plays an undeniable influence on postoperative outcomes, as does the stringent adherence to technical details. When determining the best potential bariatric intervention for a patient, the clinician must use their astute judgment and understanding of the potential complications. Gastroesophageal reflux disease is one particular comorbidity which should garner special attention as we have discussed in this chapter. Patients with a significant history of reflux should most often undergo a roux-en-Y gastric bypass as that procedure has undoubtedly shown the most reliability in resolving reflux disease. Additionally, it acts as the standard of conversion in bariatric revision cases for patients experiencing reflux symptoms after other bariatric procedures (LSG, LAGB, etc.). LSG continues to be evaluated in the light of long term follow up and remains promising. Patients with pre-existing reflux who seek a LSG should be counseled at the potential for progressively worse reflux post-operatively and a need for additional intervention to control the reflux. LSG should be used with caution in these patients. Additional long term data is needed to determine the role of endoscopic interventions in patients with reflux after bariatric surgery, though it appears this avenue of intervention will continue to expand in bariatric surgery and clinicians should remain current on newly developed technologies and techniques.

References

1. Ogden CL, Carroll MD, Fryar CD, Flegal KM. Prevalence of obesity among adults and youth: United States, 2011–2014. Washington, D.C.: US Department of Health and Human Services, Centers for Disease Control and Prevention, National Center for Health Statistics; 2015.
2. Schirmer B, Schauer P. The surgical management of obesity. In: Brunicardi FC, editor. Schwartz's principles of surgery. 9th ed. New York, NY: McGraw-Hill; 2010. p. 949–78.
3. Khorgami Z, Shoar S, Andalib A, Aminian A, Brethauer SA, Schauer PR. Trends in utilization of bariatric surgery, 2010-2014: sleeve gastrectomy dominates. Surg Obes Relat Dis. 2017;13(5):774–8.
4. Hutter MM, Schirmer BD, Jones DB, Ko CY, Cohen ME, Merkow RP, et al. First report from the American College of Surgeons Bariatric Surgery Center Network: laparoscopic sleeve gastrectomy has morbidity and effectiveness positioned between the band and the bypass. Ann Surg. 2011;254(3):410–20; discussion 420-2
5. Rrezza E, Ikramuddin S, Gourash W, Rakitt T, Kingston A, Luketich J, et al. Symptomatic improvement in gastroesophageal reflux disease (GERD) following laparoscopic Roux-en-Y gastric bypass. Surg Endosc. 2002;16(7):1027–31.
6. Casillas RA, Um SS, Getty JLZ, Sachs S, Kim BB. Revision of primary sleeve gastrectomy to Roux-en-Y gastric bypass: indications and outcomes from a high-volume center. Surg Obes Relat Dis. 2016;12(10):1817–25.
7. Schirmer B, Hallowell P. Morbid obesity and its surgical treatment. In: Maingot's abdominal operations. 12th ed. New York: McGraw-Hill; 2013. p. 545–78.
8. Iovino P, Angrisani L, Galloro G, Consalvo D, Tremolaterra F, Pascariello A, et al. Proximal stomach function in obesity with normal or abnormal oesophageal acid exposure. Neurogastroenterol Motil. 2006;18(6):425–32.
9. Emerenziani S, Rescio MP, Guarino MP, Cicala M. Gastro-esophageal reflux disease and obesity, where is the link? World J Gastroenterol. 2013;19(39):6536–9.
10. Boules M, Corcelles R, Guerron AD, Dong M, Daigle CR, El-Hayek K, et al. The incidence of hiatal hernia and technical feasibility of repair during bariatric surgery. Surgery. 2015;158(4):911–8.
11. Sharaf RN, Weinshel EH, Bini EJ, Rosenberg J, Sherman A, Ren CJ. Endoscopy plays an important preoperative role in bariatric surgery. Obes Surg. 2004;14(10):1367–72.
12. Zeni TM, Frantzides CT, Mahr C, Denham EW, Meiselman M, Goldberg MJ, et al. Value of preoperative upper endoscopy in patients undergoing laparoscopic gastric bypass. Obes Surg. 2006;16(2):142–6.
13. Oleynikov D, Ranade A, Parcells J, Bills N. Chapter 6: paraesophageal hernias and Nissen fundoplication. In: Oleynikov D, Bills N, editors. Robotic surgery for the general surgeon. 1st ed. New York: Nova Biomedical; 2014. p. 65–74.

14. Kahrilas PJ, Kim HC, Pandolfino JE. Approaches to the diagnosis and grading of hiatal hernia. Best Pract Res Clin Gastroenterol. 2008;22(4):601–16.
15. O'rourke RW, Khajanchee YS, Urbach DR, Lee NN, Lockhart B, Hansen PD, et al. Extended transmediastinal dissection: an alternative to gastroplasty for short esophagus. Arch Surg. 2003;138(7):735–40.
16. Nelson LG, Gonzalez R, Haines K, Gallagher SF, Murr MM. Amelioration of gastroesophageal reflux symptoms following Roux-en-Y gastric bypass for clinically significant obesity. Am Surg. 2005;71(11):950–4.
17. Madalosso CA, Gurski RR, Callegari-Jacques SM, Navarini D, Mazzini G, Pereira Mda S. The impact of gastric bypass on gastroesophageal reflux disease in morbidly obese patients. Ann Surg. 2016;263(1):110–6.
18. Smith SC, Edwards CB, Goodman GN. Symptomatic and clinical improvement in morbidly obese patients with gastroesophageal reflux disease following roux-en-Y gastric bypass. Obes Surg. 1997;7(6):479–84.
19. Merrouche M, Sabaté J, Jouet P, Harnois F, Scaringi S, Coffin B, et al. Gastro-esophageal reflux and esophageal motility disorders in morbidly obese patients before and after bariatric surgery. Obes Surg. 2007;17(7):894–900.
20. Korenkov M, Köhler L, Yücel N, Grass G, Troidl S, Lempa M, et al. Esophageal motility and reflux symptoms before and after bariatric surgery. Obes Surg. 2002;12(1):72–6.
21. Rebecchi F, Allaix ME, Patti MG, Schlottmann F, Morino M. Gastroesophageal reflux disease and morbid obesity: to sleeve or not to sleeve? World J Gastroenterol. 2017;23(13):2269.
22. Mattar S, Qureshi F, Taylor D, Schauer P. Treatment of refractory gastroesophageal reflux disease with radiofrequency energy (Stretta) in patients after roux-en-Y gastric bypass. Surg Endosc. 2006;20(6):850–4.
23. Carrodeguas L, Szomstein S, Soto F, Whipple O, Simpfendorfer C, Gonzalvo JP, et al. Management of gastrogastric fistulas after divided Roux-en-Y gastric bypass surgery for morbid obesity: analysis of 1292 consecutive patients and review of literature. Surg Obes Relat Dis. 2005;1(5):467–74.
24. Gumbs AA, Duffy AJ, Bell RL. Management of gastrogastric fistula after laparoscopic Roux-en-Y gastric bypass. Surg Obes Relat Dis. 2006;2(2):117–21.
25. Fernandez-Esparrach G, Lautz DB, Thompson CC. Endoscopic repair of gastrogastric fistula after Roux-en-Y gastric bypass: a less-invasive approach. Surg Obes Relat Dis. 2010;6(3):282–8.
26. Ribeiro-Parenti L, De Courville G, Daikha A, Arapis K, Chosidow D, Marmuse J. Classification, surgical management and outcomes of patients with gastrogastric fistula after Roux-En-Y gastric bypass. Surg Obes Relat Dis. 2017;13(2):243–8.
27. Poghosyan T, Caille C, Moszkowicz D, Hanachi M, Carette C, Bouillot J. Roux-en-Y gastric bypass for the treatment of severe complications after omega-loop gastric bypass. Surg Obes Relat Dis. 2017;13(6):988–94.
28. Rosenthal RJ, Panel, International Sleeve Gastrectomy Expert. International Sleeve Gastrectomy Expert Panel Consensus Statement: best practice guidelines based on experience of> 12,000 cases. Surg Obes Relat Dis. 2012;8(1):8–19.
29. Rebecchi F, Allaix ME, Giaccone C, Ugliono E, Scozzari G, Morino M. Gastroesophageal reflux disease and laparoscopic sleeve gastrectomy: a physiopathologic evaluation. Ann Surg. 2014;260(5):909–14; discussion 914-5
30. Daes J, Jimenez ME, Said N, Daza JC, Dennis R. Laparoscopic sleeve gastrectomy: symptoms of gastroesophageal reflux can be reduced by changes in surgical technique. Obes Surg. 2012;22(12):1874–9.
31. Petersen WV, Meile T, Küper MA, Zdichavsky M, Königsrainer A, Schneider JH. Functional importance of laparoscopic sleeve gastrectomy for the lower esophageal sphincter in patients with morbid obesity. Obes Surg. 2012;22(3):360–6.
32. Chiu S, Birch DW, Shi X, Sharma AM, Karmali S. Effect of sleeve gastrectomy on gastroesophageal reflux disease: a systematic review. Surg Obes Relat Dis. 2011;7(4):510–5.

33. Soricelli E, Casella G, Rizzello M, Calì B, Alessandri G, Basso N. Initial experience with laparoscopic crural closure in the management of hiatal hernia in obese patients undergoing sleeve gastrectomy. Obes Surg. 2010;20(8):1149–53.
34. Snyder B, Wilson E, Wilson T, Mehta S, Bajwa K, Klein C. A randomized trial comparing reflux symptoms in sleeve gastrectomy patients with or without hiatal hernia repair. Surg Obes Relat Dis. 2016;12(9):1681–8.
35. Iannelli A, Debs T, Martini F, Benichou B, Amor IB, Gugenheim J. Laparoscopic conversion of sleeve gastrectomy to roux-en-Y gastric bypass: indications and preliminary results. Surg Obes Relat Dis. 2016;12(8):1533–8.
36. Parmar CD, Mahawar KK, Boyle M, Schroeder N, Balupuri S, Small PK. Conversion of sleeve gastrectomy to roux-en-Y gastric bypass is effective for gastro-oesophageal reflux disease but not for further weight loss. Obes Surg. 2017;27:1–8.

Approach to Esophageal Motility Disorders

5

Alison Goldin and Wai-Kit Lo

Introduction

Esophageal motility disorders are a broad range of diseases that can present with a variety of symptoms. A careful clinical assessment can suggest the etiology, but high-resolution esophageal manometry (HREM) is the gold standard for diagnosis. Management depends on the type of motility disorder identified and ranges from medical treatment to more definitive endoscopic and surgical options.

Pathophysiology

Esophageal motility disorders result from dysfunction of one or more components of esophageal peristalsis including esophageal body contraction and lower esophageal sphincter (LES) relaxation. The smooth muscle of the esophageal body and LES are modulated by inhibitory and excitatory innervation, and the specific neurologic defect can dictate the pathologic outcome (Fig. 5.1). Inhibitory innervation, composed of preganglionic neurons in the vagus and postganglionic neurons in the myenteric plexus, results in the release of nitric oxide and vasoactive intestinal peptide, which allows for relaxation of the LES and modulates contractility in the esophageal body. When absent, disorders including achalasia (poor relaxation of the LES) and diffuse esophageal spasm (DES) (poorly modulated contraction in the esophageal body) can

A. Goldin, M.D., M.P.H.
Brigham and Women's Hospital, Harvard Medical School, Boston, MA, USA

W.-K. Lo, M.D., M.P.H. (✉)
VA Boston Healthcare System, Brigham and Women's Hospital, Harvard Medical School, Boston, MA, USA
e-mail: wlo4@partners.org

© Springer International Publishing AG, part of Springer Nature 2018
D. Oleynikov, P. M. Fisichella (eds.), *A Mastery Approach to Complex Esophageal Diseases*, https://doi.org/10.1007/978-3-319-75795-7_5

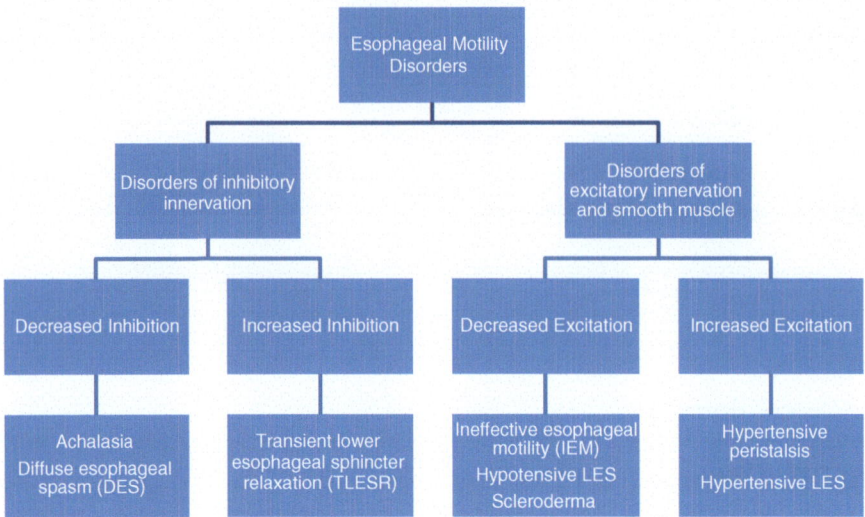

Fig. 5.1 Pathophysiologic classification of motility disorders by impact of abnormal inhibitory and excitatory innervation

result. Conversely, an increase in inhibitory innervation can result in increased transient LES relaxation (TLESR) episodes, accompanied by pathologic reflux.

Excitatory innervation, composed of vagal preganglionic and postganglionic neurons, results in the release of substance P and acetylcholine, establishing basal LES pressure and peristaltic contraction pressure. When absent, disorders including hypotensive LES, which can be associated with reflux, and hypotensive peristalsis, often seen in scleroderma, may result. Conversely, an increase in excitatory innervation may lead to disorders of hypertensive contractility, such as jackhammer esophagus.

Traditionally, motility disorders have been classified into disorders of hypocontractility (such as achalasia types I and II, and scleroderma) and hypercontractility (such as DES, jackhammer esophagus, and type III "spastic" achalasia). However, with the development of HREM and the Chicago classification to guide interpretation and diagnosis, a new organizational hierarchy for motility disorders was introduced (Fig. 5.2). Major disorders of motility are generally pathologic, and often require advanced treatments such as surgery. These include achalasia, esophagogastric junction outflow obstruction, DES, jackhammer esophagus, and absent contractility. Minor disorders of motility may not always be pathologic or result in clinical symptoms, and can include ineffective esophageal motility (IEM), fragmented peristalsis, and other less well-defined diagnoses. We will be using this framework to guide our discussion of specific motility diagnoses in the following sections.

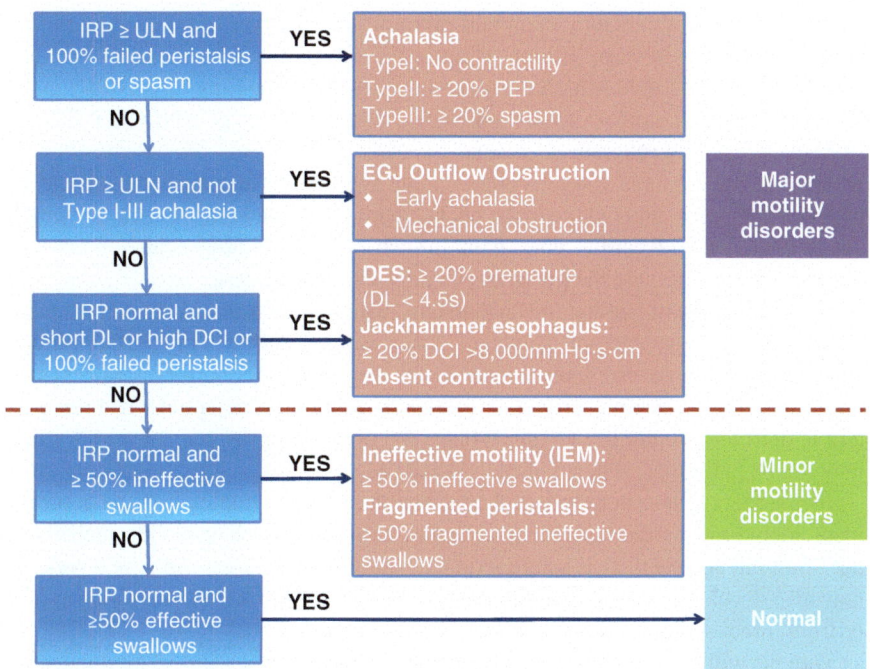

Fig. 5.2 The Chicago Classification v3.0. Esophageal motility disorders are organized by major disorders of motility (generally pathologic, including disorders of EGJ obstruction with poor LES relaxation), and minor disorders of motility (which can be a normal variant). *IRP* integrated relaxation pressure, *ULN* upper limit of normal, *PEP* pan-esophageal pressurization, *DL* distal latency, *DCI* distal contractile integral

Clinical Assessment

The clinical symptoms of patients with esophageal motility disorders depend upon the etiology. Symptoms range from dysphagia to chest pain. Dysphagia to solids and liquids, consisting of a sensation of food or liquid lodged in the esophagus after initiation of a normal swallow, is one of the most common symptoms. Patients often feel that the bolus is hung up at the level of the suprasternal notch, although this may not be reflective of the actual location of the impacted food or liquid bolus. Learned behaviors to aid in swallowing and compensate for symptoms include taking longer to eat a meal, drinking fluids to clear food from the esophagus, eating smaller amounts of food, and performing physical maneuvers such as standing or arching the back to enhance bolus passage. Weight loss is common, and an indication for expedited evaluation. Other possible symptoms include chest pain or discomfort and/or regurgitation of liquid or food bolus.

In achalasia, patients may complain of vomit that dribbles out onto their pillow overnight. The main complication of untreated achalasia is the eventual development of megaesophagus, which is irreversible. There is also a small risk of developing squamous cell cancer of the esophagus, although there is insufficient data to support a screening program at present.

In DES, chest pain is often the predominant symptom. This pain can be triggered by emotional stress and radiate to the back, lateral chest and both arms or jaw, which can be confused with cardiac chest pain. In such cases, cardiology evaluation should be prioritized to exclude the presence of cardiovascular disease.

In hypertensive or jackhammer esophagus, patients often complain of chest pain, in addition to or in place of dysphagia. Interestingly, episodes of high-amplitude contractions seen on esophageal manometry do not always correlate with symptoms, and can be a normal variant, so clinical correlation is essential when this pattern is detected on motility testing. This is the only major disorder of motility that may not be pathologic when detected on HREM.

In disorders of absent esophageal contractility, GERD symptoms are most prominent, including heartburn, dysphagia, regurgitation, and chest pain. One such disorder of absent contractility is scleroderma, an autoimmune disease in which patients may also develop concomitant pulmonary interstitial fibrosis from micro-aspiration or from direct scleroderma involvement of lung tissue.

Patients with minor disorders of motility may complain of reflux symptoms or no symptoms at all. Clinical correlation is required when these findings are seen on HREM.

Diagnostic Procedures

Upper endoscopy is generally required in patients with suspected esophageal motility disorders to rule out mechanical causes, including stricture and malignancy. This is especially important in patients presenting with alarm symptoms including dysphagia or weight loss. Additionally, biopsies of the mid- and distal esophagus should be obtained to rule out eosinophilic esophagitis, an inflammatory condition causing dysphagia which occurs when eosinophils infiltrate the esophageal mucosa. Esophageal biopsies may also evaluate for evidence of infectious esophagitis, including HSV and candida, which is in the differential diagnosis of dysphagia. In achalasia, upper endoscopy is important to rule out gastroesophageal junction tumors, which can result in secondary achalasia.

Laboratory testing can be used to support manometric diagnoses. In achalasia, antibodies to the parasite *T. cruzi* should be considered in patients with risk factors, such as foreign travel, to evaluate for secondary achalasia due to parasitic infection. Additionally, antineuronal antibodies should be checked when paraneoplastic syndromes are suspected as the cause of secondary achalasia, particularly in patients with small cell cancers of the breast or lung. In scleroderma, antibody testing to topoisomerase-1 (Scl 70) can provide additional support for the diagnosis.

Radiologic studies can also be useful in the assessment of motility disorders. Barium swallow may demonstrate classic "bird-beaking" of the lower esophagus in achalasia, or a corkscrew appearance of the esophagus in DES. In advanced achalasia, the esophagus may appear sigmoid with severe dilation and an acute angle in the distal esophagus, or feature evidence of an esophageal diverticulum. There may also be delayed emptying and impaired or absent peristalsis of the esophagus noted as part of the study, which may be a more general signifier of dyskinesia. Chest imaging may be used in achalasia to exclude secondary achalasia due to pulmonary malignancy.

Multichannel intraluminal impedance and pH (MII-pH) testing may be helpful to evaluate for contribution from acid or bolus reflux. Some motility disorders, such as scleroderma, often co-present with reflux symptoms. Other findings, such as IEM, are frequently detected in the presence of GERD, and are often associated with evidence of increased reflux on MII-pH testing.

The gold standard for diagnosis of esophageal motility disorders is HREM. This diagnostic tool measures esophageal peristalsis, baseline LES pressure and relaxation, and bolus transit. Esophageal manometry involves placement of a thin flexible catheter with sequential pressure sensors transnasally into the stomach, traversing the esophagus and LES in the process. Patients are asked to take ten swallows with 5 mL of water in the supine position, and in some centers, an additional ten swallows with thick gel is also performed. Recently, as mentioned above, the Chicago classification was proposed to provide an organizational scheme for the diagnosis of motility disorders, dividing them into major and minor disorders based on manometric parameters [1]. This classification system allows for greater standardization in the diagnosis and classification of motility disorders. The Chicago parameters include the distal contractile integral (DCI), distal latency (DL), contractile deceleration point (CDP), and integrated relaxation pressure (IRP) (Table 5.1, Figs. 5.2 and 5.3). The DCI is the product of the mean amplitude of contraction in the distal esophagus (mmHg), duration of contraction (seconds), and the length of the distal esophageal segment (cm)—essentially a measure of distal

Table 5.1 Definitions and threshold values of high resolution esophageal manometry parameters referenced in the Chicago classification of motility disorders

Metric	Definition
Integrated relaxation pressure (IRP)	Measure of LES relaxation *Abnormal*: >15 mmHg, or higher depending on HREM machine model
Distal latency (DL)	Measure of esophageal spasm/spontaneous swallow *Abnormal*: <4.5 s
Distal contractile integral (DCI)	Measure of distal esophageal contractile force *Failed*: <100 mmHg·s·cm *Weak*: 100–450 mmHg·s·cm *Normal*: 450–8000 mmHg·s·cm *Hypertensive*: >8000 mmHg·s·cm

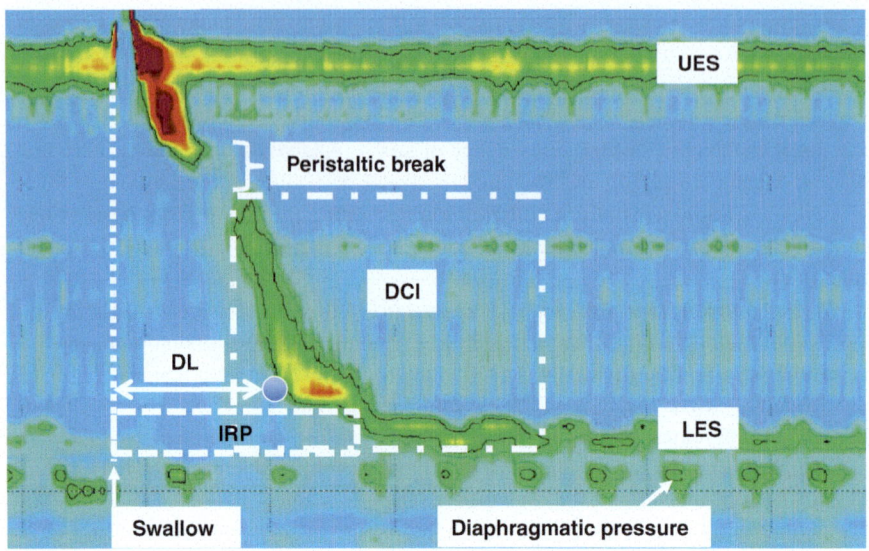

Fig. 5.3 Chicago Classification Parameters on High Resolution Esophageal Manometry. The blue dot signifies the contractile deceleration point (CDP). *UES* upper esophageal sphincter, *DCI* distal contractile integral, *DL* distal latency, *IRP* integrated relaxation pressure, *LES* lower esophageal sphincter

esophageal contractile force. It is considered failed if less than 100 mmHg·s·cm, weak if less than 450 mmHg·s·cm, and hypercontractile if greater than 8000 mmHg·s·cm. DL is measured from the time of upper esophageal sphincter relaxation to an inflection in the peristaltic axis, or CDP, and is considered premature if less than 4.5 s. DL is a measure of esophageal spasm. The IRP is measured as the mean EGJ pressure during the 4 s of maximal relaxation in the first 10 s after upper esophageal sphincter relaxation, relative to gastric baseline, and is considered elevated if greater than 15 mmHg, though this cutoff is dependent on the model of HREM machine. IRP is a measure of LES relaxation.

The first two diagnoses in the Chicago classification hierarchy are ones in which the median IRP is elevated, reflecting poor LES relaxation.

HREM is a sensitive method to diagnose achalasia [2]. Manometric parameters that meet criteria for achalasia include median IRP >15 mmHg across all swallows, with 100% failed peristalsis or esophageal spasm. HREM allows for achalasia to be classified into three subtypes based on the pattern of contractility in the esophagus, with implications for treatment success. Type I "classic" achalasia is defined by failed contractions without esophageal pressurization. Type II achalasia is characterized by aperistalsis with pan-esophageal pressurization. Type III "spastic" achalasia is defined by high amplitude spastic or premature contractions [1]. Type II achalasia is the most common subtype and is most responsive to treatment, whereas type III achalasia is the least common subtype and is also the least treatment responsive.

Esophagogastric junction outflow obstruction (EGJOO) is characterized manometrically by impaired LES relaxation with median IRP >15 mmHg but normal or weak peristalsis. In some cases, this may reflect incompletely expressed achalasia, and should be monitored closely. It is also important to exclude mechanical obstruction.

The next three diagnoses feature normal IRP, accompanied by other abnormal parameters.

DES is characterized manometrically by a normal IRP, but with simultaneous, non-peristaltic contractions featuring DL less than 4.5 s, in at least 20% of swallows. The non-peristaltic contractions are due to loss of inhibitory nerve function in the esophagus, similar to achalasia, and the contractions themselves can have either increased or decreased amplitudes. One distinguishing feature from Type III achalasia is that with DES, the lower esophageal sphincter is spared and relaxes normally.

Hypertensive esophagus, or "jackhammer" esophagus, is characterized manometrically by a normal IRP and normal DL, but with a DCI greater than 8000 in at least 20% of swallows.

Absent contractility is defined by normal IRP with evidence of aperistalsis. It encompasses diagnoses such as scleroderma, which is not a distinct diagnosis in the Chicago classification. Hypotensive LES may also be seen in scleroderma.

The preceding diagnoses are considered major disorders of peristalsis, which are generally pathologic.

Minor disorders of peristalsis include IEM defined by greater than 50% failed or weak swallows, and fragmented peristalsis defined by greater than 50% contractions with peristaltic breaks of at least 5 cm. These findings are not always clinically significant, so clinical correlation is recommended before pursuing treatment.

Treatment Options

Achalasia

Treatment ranges from pharmacologic therapy, to endoscopic and surgical interventions, which are more invasive but also more effective. The goal of therapy for all approaches is to decrease the resting LES pressure, allowing for passage of solids and liquids into the stomach. Overall, treatment response is highest for patients with Type II achalasia.

Pharmacologic Options
Medical therapy has limited efficacy in the treatment of achalasia. In patients who cannot tolerate any endoscopic or surgical intervention, nitrates and calcium channel blockers may be used to decrease LES pressure to enhance bolus clearance. However, these medications tend to be short-acting, with maximum pharmacologic duration of 120 min, and are often limited by side effects including dizziness and headaches [3]. Thus, medical therapy should be avoided as long as endoscopic or surgical options remain viable.

Endoscopic Botulinum Toxin Injection

Botulinum toxin A (Botox) inhibits acetylcholine release. When injected into the LES, it lowers LES pressure. Approximately 25 units of Botox total are injected into the four quadrants of the LES. Initial response rates are high at 80%, but the effect seems to be transient, with many patients requiring repeat injections with diminished efficacy over time [4–6]. This may be due to antibody formation to the toxin as well as fibrosis of the LES from repeated treatments. In spite of this, Botox does benefit from minimal side effects and ease of delivery, and is therefore most often reserved for non-surgical candidates with achalasia, such as elderly patients.

Pneumatic Dilation

Pneumatic dilation uses air filled balloons under high pressure to mechanically disrupt the smooth muscle of the distal esophagus and LES. The dilators typically range in size from 30 to 40 mm. Pneumatic dilation is performed using fluoroscopic guidance with the balloon crossing the LES. Usually two or more dilations are required, resulting in high remission rates at 1–5 years after treatment. Four percent of dilations cause perforations requiring surgical repair, which is more common in patients requiring serial dilations compared to single dilation [7]. Perforation, though rare, is more frequent with balloons greater then 30 mm, and with the initial dilation [8]. Relapse is more likely to occur in males, subjects with extreme esophageal dilatation, younger age (<40), and poor bolus emptying on timed barium swallow [7, 9, 10]. Because pneumatic dilation is less invasive than myotomy, it is often the preferred approach in subjects with surgical risk factors, such as older age and medical comorbidities.

Heller Myotomy

First performed in 1913, the Heller myotomy is now performed laparoscopically and usually with an extended myotomy into the cardia of the stomach. The extended myotomy allows for further reduction of LES pressures to a goal of <10 mmHg. However, this comes at the risk of significant reflux. To help mitigate this risk, a partial fundoplication (either anterior Dor with 180° wrap, or posterior Toupet with 270° wrap) is also performed [11, 12]. Symptomatic improvement occurs in 90% of patients post-operatively, though efficacy does decrease with time [4]. The most common complication is GERD requiring PPI treatment in upwards of 40% of patients, even when a partial wrap is performed. However, a complete wrap or Nissen fundoplication is usually avoided, since it can become difficult to distinguish post-operative dysphagia from a tight wrap versus an incomplete myotomy. In certain cases of Type III achalasia, the myotomy can be extended proximally in the esophagus to address severe esophageal spasticity.

Laparoscopic Heller myotomy is superior to a single pneumatic dilation but this difference dissipates with graded pneumatic dilations guided by clinical symptoms. A meta-analysis comparing graded pneumatic dilation to laparoscopic myotomy determined myotomy was more effective than pneumatic dilation, but there were no differences in reflux rates and LES pressure [13]. The largest trial included in the meta-analysis found no significant difference in success rate for pneumatic dilation

(90%) versus Heller myotomy (93%) at 1 year [14]. Five years after treatment, there remained no significant difference in success rates between the myotomy and pneumatic dilation groups [15].

Endoscopic Myotomy

Per-oral endoscopic myotomy (POEM) is a newer alterative to surgical myotomy. It is a form of natural orifice transluminal endoscopic surgery (NOTES). This is an incisionless surgery performed with a flexible endoscope, with submucosal tunneling made distal to the mucosal incision. Contraindications include severe esophagitis, coagulation disorders, prior therapy with possible submucosal fibrosis such as radiation, endoscopic mucosal resection, and portal hypertension. The technique involves four steps: (1) mucosal incision with entry into the submucosa, (2) formation of a submucosal tunnel, (3) myotomy, and (4) closure of the mucosal incision. In POEM, the circular muscle of the LES is disrupted and the longitudinal muscle layer is left intact. The technique involves insertion of a flexible endoscope into the esophagus and use of a very small electrosurgical knife through the instrument channel of the endoscopy. A small mucosal incision is made in the mid esophagus so that the endoscope can then enter into the 1–2 mm submucosal space between the mucosa and muscularis propria. This space is expanded with saline injections to provide space for insertion of the 10-mm endoscope, which is subsequently advanced to create a tunnel into the gastric cardia. A myotomy is then performed within the tunnel. The length of the myotomy depends upon the underlying disorder and is typically longer in spastic esophageal disorders compared to achalasia subtype I or II. Finally the original mucosal incision is closed with sutures or endoscopic clips [16]. Typically patients are admitted to the hospital overnight for observation and given prophylactic antibiotics and antiemetics. An esophagram is obtained the day after the procedure to rule out an esophageal leak and the diet is advanced to a soft diet for the next 2 weeks. POEM is a safe procedure with low rates of adverse events which include pneumoperitoneum, pneumothorax, bleeding, mucosal perforation and gastroesophageal reflux (which is of concern since a partial fundoplication cannot be performed at the time of POEM unlike during laparoscopic Heller myotomy). POEM has demonstrated a high rate of clinical success (82–100%) and is comparable to laparoscopic Heller myotomy in safety and efficacy based on a recent meta-analysis [17]. POEM is also effective and safe in patients who have refractory or recurrent symptoms despite prior surgical or endoscopic treatment [18].

EGJ Outflow Obstruction

There are no specific treatments for EGJOO since the etiology of this entity is not well understood. It may be a variant of or represent early achalasia. Alternatively, it may be caused by abnormal anatomy at the cardia including a hiatal hernia. The same treatment options available for achalasia may be applied for EGJOO. However, as many as one-third of patients diagnosed with EGJOO experience spontaneous symptom resolution without specific intervention. Medical therapies such as calcium channel blockers and nitrates may be used, but only 50% of patients experience a response [19]. More invasive treatment options including Botox injection, pneumatic dilation, or surgery are all highly efficacious with favorable outcomes, but given the unclear natural history of this diagnosis, are reserved for severe cases. Recently, the use of acotiamide hydrochloride, a prokinetic drug approved for functional dyspepsia, may offer some treatment benefit in EGJOO. Acotiamide acts as an acetylcholinesterase inhibitor with prokinetic activity and improved gastric emptying, and 83.3% of EGJOO patients reported at least some symptomatic improvement as well as normalization of the IRP following its use [20–22].

Diffuse Esophageal Spasm

Treatment of DES can be difficult and therapy is mainly focused on symptom control, primarily because of the current lack of understanding of the underlying etiology of DES and dearth of controlled therapeutic trials. Proton pump inhibitors and histamine receptor antagonists may be used to address any contribution from acid reflux, which has the potential to induce or be a consequence of esophageal spasm. Smooth muscle relaxants including nitrates and calcium channel blockers, anticholinergics, and phosphodiesterase-5 inhibitors are used to decrease LES pressure and esophageal contraction amplitude. While nitrates have not been tested in a controlled fashion in patients with DES or other spastic disorders, they have been demonstrated manometrically to prolong the DL and decrease distal contraction amplitude [23]. Phosphodiesterase-5 inhibitors such as sildenafil block the breakdown of nitric oxide and thereby prolong smooth muscle relaxation [24]. Many of these therapies are limited by side effects such as headache and dizziness. Low dose antidepressants (tricyclic antidepressants, serotonin receptor inhibitors, trazodone) are effective in improving chest pain caused by DES, though data does not demonstrate any effect on motility. This suggests that visceral hypersensitivity could be a major driver of symptoms [25]. Studies have demonstrated that more invasive techniques such as empiric bougie dilation or Botox injection of the LES alone do not significantly improve symptoms, though data is more promising when considering Botox injection of the esophageal body [26, 27]. Pneumatic dilation, while effective in the treatment of achalasia, has not been proven in DES. Limited data demonstrates some improvement with an extended Heller myotomy, but this invasive approach is reserved for refractory patients [28]. A recent systematic review and meta-analysis demonstrated POEM as an effective and safe treatment modality for spastic esophageal disorders including type III achalasia, diffuse esophageal spasm and jackhammer esophagus [29].

Overall, treatment of DES should be approached in a stepwise fashion. First, the patient should be placed on antireflux medication. If this therapy is ineffective, a smooth muscle relaxant such as a calcium channel blocker or a treatment for visceral hypersensitivity such as tricyclic antidepressant can be tried. If symptoms persist, more invasive treatments such as Botox injection can be considered. Finally, surgery is reserved for patients who fail all other treatment modalities.

Hypercontractile (Jackhammer) Esophagus

Similar to DES, therapy of hypercontractile esophagus is aimed at symptom control, as the underlying pathophysiology remains poorly understood. Treatment is dictated by the predominant clinical complaint. Smooth muscle relaxants including nitrates and calcium channel blockers, as well as anticholinergic medications, may be applied to treat symptoms of dysphagia. For subjects with noncardiac chest pain, tricyclic antidepressants may help address the clinical contribution from visceral hypersensitivity. In severe cases, Botox injection in the esophageal body has resulted in clinical improvement in dysphagia symptoms and may be an option for select patients [27].

Absent Peristalsis/Scleroderma Esophagus

The current treatment of absent esophageal peristalsis includes aggressive reflux management, with use of proton pump inhibitors at maximum dose. Unfortunately, prokinetic medications have not demonstrated clinical utility in this patient population. Scleroderma esophagus is a connective tissue disorder that affects the smooth muscle of the esophagus, resulting in aperistalsis and decreased LES pressure. Antireflux surgery has been discouraged because of the risk of significant postoperative dysphagia with decreased or absent peristalsis of the esophageal body, although some studies have proposed partial fundoplication to manage severe GERD symptoms in select patients with absent peristalsis [30]. Esophageal strictures may develop from significant uncontrolled reflux and often require dilation.

Ineffective Esophageal Motility

Treatment options are limited for IEM. Because most cases are associated with GERD, treatment is aimed at antireflux control. Buspirone is a serotonin receptor agonist which may enhance LES resting pressure in IEM, and presents a possible treatment for IEM regardless of reflux association, in patients with clinical symptoms of dysphagia [31].

Fragmented Peristalsis

Similar to IEM, treatment options are limited in fragmented peristalsis because the clinical implications of this diagnosis remain unclear. Treatment tends to be focused on management of concomitant GERD.

Summary

Esophageal motility disorders are a broad category of diseases with a variety of symptoms, including dysphagia and chest pain. The pathophysiology is not always fully understood, but may involve alterations in inhibitory or excitatory innervation of the smooth muscle of the distal esophagus and LES. The gold standard in diagnosis is HREM, and the Chicago classification offers an organizational framework for better evaluation and management. Major disorders of motility are generally pathologic, and include achalasia, EGJOO, DES, hypertensive esophagus, and absent peristalsis, such as scleroderma. Minor disorders including IEM may be associated with GERD or have no clinical correlation. Treatments are targeted at the particular diagnosis. In achalasia, endoscopic and surgical options are preferred. For the remaining motility diagnoses, medical management forms the mainstay of treatment, which can be limited by side effect profiles.

References

1. Kahrilas PJ, Bredenoord AJ, Fox M, et al. The Chicago classification of esophageal motility disorders, v3.0. Neurogastroenterol Motil. 2015;27(2):160–74. https://doi.org/10.1111/nmo.12477.
2. Richter JE. High-resolution manometry in diagnosis and treatment of achalasia: help or hype. Curr Gastroenterol Rep. 2015;17(1):420. https://doi.org/10.1007/s11894-014-0420-2.
3. Hoogerwerf WA, Pasricha PJ. Pharmacologic therapy in treating achalasia. Gastrointest Endosc Clin N Am. 2001;11(2):311–24, vii. http://www.ncbi.nlm.nih.gov/pubmed/11319064
4. Campos GM, Vittinghoff E, Rabl C, et al. Endoscopic and surgical treatments for achalasia: a systematic review and meta-analysis. Ann Surg. 2009;249(1):45–57. https://doi.org/10.1097/SLA.0b013e31818e43ab.
5. Fishman VM, Parkman HP, Schiano TD, et al. Symptomatic improvement in achalasia after botulinum toxin injection of the lower esophageal sphincter. Am J Gastroenterol. 1996;91(9):1724–30. http://ovidsp.ovid.com/ovidweb.cgi?T=JS&PAGE=reference&D=med4&NEWS=N&AN=8792688
6. Annese V, Bassotti G, Coccia G, et al. A multicentre randomised study of intrasphincteric botulinum toxin in patients with oesophageal achalasia. GISMAD Achalasia Study Group. Gut. 2000;46(5):597–600. https://doi.org/10.1136/gut.46.5.597.
7. Katzka DA, Castell DO. Review article: an analysis of the efficacy, perforation rates and methods used in pneumatic dilation for achalasia. Aliment Pharmacol Ther. 2011;34(8):832–9. https://doi.org/10.1111/j.1365-2036.2011.04816.x.
8. Richter JE, Vela MF, Richter JE, et al. Update on the management of achalasia: balloons, surgery and drugs. Clin Gastroenterol Hepatol. 2006;4(3):580–7. https://doi.org/10.1586/17474124.2.3.435.
9. Eckardt VF, Aignherr C, Bernhard G. Predictors of outcome in patients with achalasia treated by pneumatic dilation. Gastroenterology. 1992;103(6):1732–8. https://doi.org/10.1053/j.gastro.2008.07.022.Achalasia.
10. Chan KC, Wong SKH, Lee DWH, et al. Short-term and long-term results of endoscopic balloon dilation for achalasia: 12 years' experience. Endoscopy. 2004;36:690–4. https://doi.org/10.1055/s-2004-825659.
11. Richards WO, Torquati A, Holzman MD, et al. Heller myotomy versus Heller myotomy with Dor fundoplication for achalasia: a prospective randomized double-blind clinical trial. Ann Surg. 2004;240(3):405–15. https://doi.org/10.1097/01.sla.0000202000.01069.4d.

12. Oelschlager BK, Chang L, Pellegrini CA. Improved outcome after extended gastric myotomy for achalasia. Arch Surg. 2003;138(5):490–495-497. https://doi.org/10.1001/archsurg.138.5.490.
13. Yaghoobi M, Mayrand S, Martel M, Roshan-Afshar I, Bijarchi R, Barkun A. Laparoscopic Heller's myotomy versus pneumatic dilation in the treatment of idiopathic achalasia: a meta-analysis of randomized, controlled trials. Gastrointest Endosc. 2013;78(3):468–75. https://doi.org/10.1016/j.gie.2013.03.1335.
14. JCY W. Pneumatic dilation versus laparoscopic Heller's myotomy for idiopathic achalasia. J Neurogastroenterol Motil. 2011;17(3):324–6. https://doi.org/10.5056/jnm.2011.17.3.324.
15. Moonen A, Annese V, Belmans A, et al. Long-term results of the European achalasia trial: a multicentre randomised controlled trial comparing pneumatic dilation versus laparoscopic Heller myotomy. Gut. 2016;65:732–9. https://doi.org/10.1136/gutjnl-2015-310602.
16. Inoue H, Minami H, Kobayashi Y, et al. Peroral endoscopic myotomy (POEM) for esophageal achalasia. Endoscopy. 2010;42(4):265–71. https://doi.org/10.1055/s-0029-1244080.
17. Marano L, Pallabazzer G, Solito B, et al. Surgery or peroral esophageal myotomy for achalasia. Medicine (Baltimore). 2016;95(10):e3001. https://doi.org/10.1097/MD.0000000000003001.
18. Stavropoulos SN, Modayil RJ, Friedel D, Savides T. The international per oral endoscopic myotomy survey (IPOEMS): a snapshot of the global POEM experience. Surg Endosc. 2013;27(9):3322–38. https://doi.org/10.1007/s00464-013-2913-8.
19. Pérez-Fernández MT, Santander C, Marinero A, Burgos-Santamaría D, Chavarría-Herbozo C. Characterization and follow-up of esophagogastric junction outflow obstruction detected by high resolution manometry. Neurogastroenterol Motil. 2016;28(1):116–26. https://doi.org/10.1111/nmo.12708.
20. Ishimura N, Mori M, Mikami H, et al. Effects of acotiamide on esophageal motor function and gastroesophageal reflux in healthy volunteers. BMC Gastroenterol. 2015;15(1):1–8. https://doi.org/10.1186/s12876-015-0346-7.
21. Kusunoki H, Haruma K, Manabe N, et al. Therapeutic efficacy of acotiamide in patients with functional dyspepsia based on enhanced postprandial gastric accommodation and emptying: randomized controlled study evaluation by real-time ultrasonography. Neurogastroenterol Motil. 2012;24(6):e250–1. https://doi.org/10.1111/j.1365-2982.2012.01897.x.
22. Muta K, Ihara E, Fukaura K, Tsuchida O, Ochiai T, Nakamura K. Effects of acotiamide on the esophageal motility function in patients with esophageal motility disorders: a pilot study. Digestion. 2016;94:9–16.
23. Konturek JW, Gillessen A, Domschke W. Diffuse esophageal spasm: a malfunction that involves nitric oxide? Scand J Gastroenterol. 1995;30(11):1041–5. https://doi.org/10.3109/00365529509101604.
24. Eherer AJ, Schwetz I, Hammer HF, et al. Effect of sildenafil on oesophageal motor function in healthy subjects and patients with oesophageal motor disorders. Gut. 2002;50(6):758–64. https://doi.org/10.1136/gut.50.6.758.
25. Hershcovici T, Achem SR, Jha LK, Fass R. Systematic review: the treatment of noncardiac chest pain. Aliment Pharmacol Ther. 2012;35(1):5–14. https://doi.org/10.1111/j.1365-2036.2011.04904.x.
26. Bashashati M, Andrews C, Ghosh S, Storr M. Botulinum toxin in the treatment of diffuse esophageal spasm. Dis Esophagus. 2010;23(7):554–60. https://doi.org/10.1111/j.1442-2050.2010.01065.x.
27. Vanuytsel T, Bisschops R, Farre R, et al. Botulinum toxin reduces dysphagia in patients with nonachalasia primary esophageal motility disorders. Clin Gastroenterol Hepatol. 2013;11(9):1115–21.e2. https://doi.org/10.1016/j.cgh.2013.03.021.
28. Leconte M, Douard R, Gaudric M, Dumontier I, Chaussade S, Dousset B. Functional results after extended myotomy for diffuse oesophageal spasm. Br J Surg. 2007;94(9):1113–8. https://doi.org/10.1002/bjs.5761.
29. Khan MA, Kumbhari V, Ngamruengphong S, et al. Is POEM the answer for management of spastic esophageal disorders? A systematic review and meta-analysis. Dig Dis Sci. 2017;62(1):35–44. https://doi.org/10.1007/s10620-016-4373-1.

30. Lund RJ, Wetcher GH, Raiser F, et al. Laparoscopic Toupet fundoplication for gastroesophageal reflux disease with poor esophageal body motility. J Gastrointest Surg. 1997;1(4):301–8.
31. Scheerens C, Tack J, Rommel N. Buspirone, a new drug for the management of patients with ineffective esophageal motility? United European Gastroenterol J. 2015;3(3):261–5. https://doi.org/10.1177/2050640615585688.

Treatment Modalities for Achalasia

6

Omar Y. Mousa, Bhaumik Brahmbhatt,
and Timothy A. Woodward

Abbreviations

ARM	Anti-reflux mucosectomy
EGD	Esophagogastroduodenoscopy
EGJ	Esophagogastric junction
GERD	Gastroesophageal reflux
HRM	High resolution manometry
IQR	Interquartile range
IRP	Integrated relaxation pressure
LES	Lower esophageal sphincter
LHM	Laparoscopic Heller myotomy
PD	Pneumatic dilation
PIVI	Preservation and incorporation of valuable endoscopic innovations
POEM	Peroral esophageal myotomy
PPI	Proton pump inhibitors
RCT	Randomized controlled trial

Introduction

Esophageal achalasia, is an uncommon esophageal motility disorder, with an incidence of 1/100,000 individuals per year and prevalence of 10/100,000. There is no gender or racial predilection and the peak incidence occurs between the third and the sixth decades of life. The disease may stem from an autoimmune,

O. Y. Mousa, M.D. · B. Brahmbhatt, M.D. · T. A. Woodward, M.D. (✉)
Division of Gastroenterology and Hepatology, Mayo Clinic, Jacksonville, FL, USA
e-mail: woodward.timothy@mayo.edu

© Springer International Publishing AG, part of Springer Nature 2018
D. Oleynikov, P. M. Fisichella (eds.), *A Mastery Approach to Complex Esophageal Diseases*, https://doi.org/10.1007/978-3-319-75795-7_6

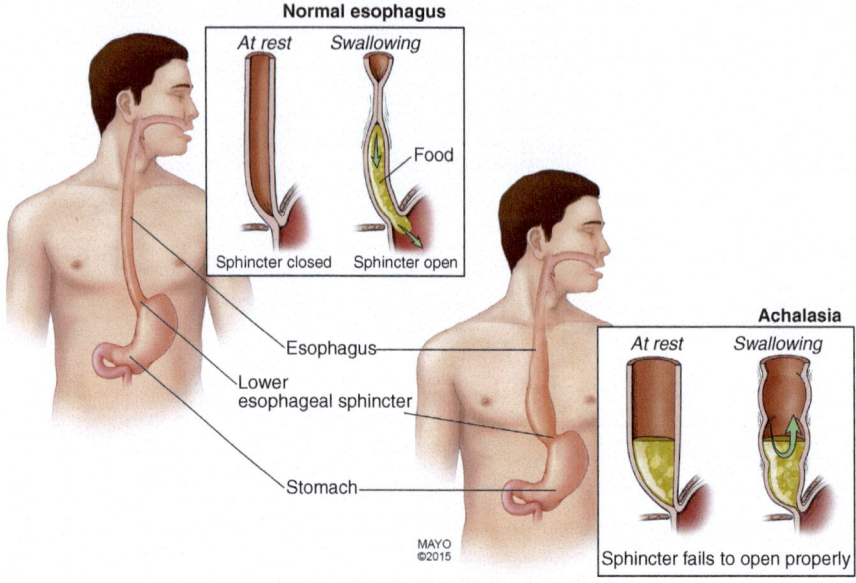

Fig. 6.1 Comparison of a normal esophagus to an esophagus with achalasia

viral or neurodegenerative process [1, 2]. Achalasia is characterized by failure of relaxation of the lower esophageal sphincter (LES) and the absence of progressive peristalsis in the distal esophagus, as shown in Fig. 6.1. In addition, intraluminal pressure in the esophagus may not be completely absent and, accordingly, patients with achalasia may have panesophageal pressurization or spastic contractions [3, 4].

Achalasia is incurable, yet a variety of treatment options are available and are capable of relieving the outflow obstruction at the esophagogastric junction (EGJ) [4]. This chapter will discuss the pathophysiology, clinical presentation, diagnosis and endoscopic evaluation and treatment of achalasia.

Pathophysiology and Clinical Presentation

Achalasia is associated with a functional loss of inhibitory postganglionic neurons of the myenteric plexus in the distal esophagus and LES [5]. It is postulated that the mechanism behind the loss is inflammatory. Nitric oxide and vasoactive intestinal peptide, normally acting as neurotransmitters, lose their inhibitory function in the setting of achalasia. The resulting imbalance leads to unopposed cholinergic stimulation, resulting in impaired relaxation of the lower esophageal sphincter and hypercontractility of the distal esophagus. There is variability in presentation of these abnormalities, though impaired relaxation of the LES is the ultimate defining feature.

Patients with esophageal achalasia classically presents with regurgitation and dysphagia to both solids and liquids. Chest pain and weight loss are common as is heartburn. Achalasia, in fact, should be considered in the differential diagnosis of patients with gastroesophageal reflux (GERD) refractory to H2 blockers and proton pump inhibitors [6]. Finally, respiratory symptoms are be frequently encountered in patients with achalasia due to the decrease clearance of contents from the esophagus secondary to the primary motor abnormality.

Diagnosis

The main diagnostic procedures used when evaluating a patient with suspected achalasia include esophageal manometry, along with two complimentary tests, esophageal radiography (esophagram) and esophagogastroduodenoscopy (EGD) [4].

It is important to note that there are diseases that may mimic achalasia in its evaluation. These include pseudoachalasia, secondary achalasia and achalasia due to Chagas disease. EGJ adenocarcinoma comprises the most common malignancies of pseudoachalasia, along with pancreas, esophagus, lung, kidney, hepatobililary, lymphoma and mesothelioma. Secondary achalasia should be considered following fundoplication surgery or gastric banding due to the development of scar tissue or an overly tight fundic wrap [7, 8].

Radiography

An esophagram will demonstrate esophageal dilation, aperistalsis, and a "bird beak" appearance due to EGJ narrowing and decreased emptying of the contrast material (Fig. 6.2). It may also reveal a tortuous or "sigmoid" esophagus which is seen in end-stage achalasia. "megaesophagus or sigmoid esophagus", which is tortuous esophagus seen in end-stage achalasia. Esophagrams are essential for posttreatment follow up [4]. Obtaining a timed barium esophagram in this instance can help identify patients who are likely to eventually fail treatment despite early improvement in their symptoms [5].

Endoscopy

Endoscopic evaluation of achalasia is important in patients who undergo EGD for the assessment of GERD. It is crucial to rule out other causes of compromised relaxation of the EGJ or abnormal contractility of the esophageal body, as in mechanical obstruction or pseudoachalasia due to infiltrating malignancy [4, 6].

Endoscopy may demonstrate normal appearing esophagus, dilated esophagus, esophagitis with ulcers secondary to stasis or candida esophagitis. The EGJ may have the appearance of a thickened muscular ring and the endoscopist may face resistance as he attempts to enter the stomach [4]. In addition, esophageal biopsies

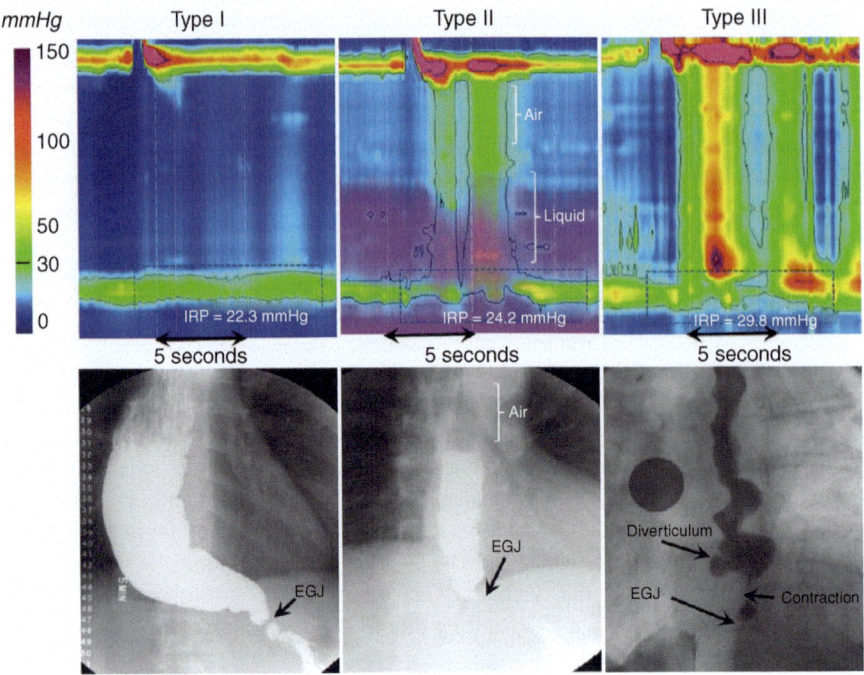

Fig. 6.2 High resolution manometry and Esophagram images comparing the three subtypes of achalasia [3]. *With permission from the Esophageal Center at Northwestern – John E. Pandolfino, MD*

in a patient with achalasia may show eosinophilia that responds to corticosteroids. This can be confused with eosinophilic esophagitis, making the presentation more complex. However, manometry along with the presenting symptoms of dysphagia can help differentiate achalasia from eosinophilic esophagitis [4, 7].

Esophageal Manometry

Esophageal manometry is essential in the diagnosis of achalasia. Esophageal manometry confirms the absence of peristalsis and incomplete relaxation of LES while excluding mechanical obstruction. Other findings that support the diagnosis include: elevated baseline pressures of the LES or the esophageal body or absence of simultaneous propagating contractile activity. This can be presented using the conventional manometry line tracing format or using esophageal pressure topography (high resolution manometry) [2].

In 2009, the Chicago Classification was first published to categorize esophageal motility disorders in high resolution manometry (HRM) using color pressure topography plots [8]. This classification was updated in 2011 and 2014 by the International HRM Working Group, to formulate version 3.0 of the Chicago Classification of esophageal motility disorders. It describes three subtypes of achalasia.

HRM tracings and esophagrams comparing the three subtypes of achalasia are shown in Fig. 6.2. Comparison is based on non-peristaltic contractility of the esophageal body and pressurization along with elevated integrated relaxation pressure (IRP) [3, 9]:

1. Type I achalasia (classic achalasia): Characterized by 100% absent peristalsis and no apparent esophageal contractility with elevated IRP > 10 mmHg. IRP is less than type II and III as there is no panpressurization of the esophagus.
   Esophagram shows dilated esophagus.
2. Type II achalasia (with esophageal compression): Abnormal relaxation of the EGJ with panesophageal pressurization that occurs with at least 20% of swallows (IRP > 30 mmHg).
   Esophagram findings correlate with manometry; air filling the proximal esophagus and liquid filling the distal esophagus.
3. Type III achalasia (spastic): Impaired EGJ relaxation and spastic contractions. To establish the diagnosis at least two swallows should be associated with a contraction that has distal latency <4.5 s. In addition, panesophageal pressurization, absent peristalsis or rapid contractions can be seen.
   Esophagram shows esophageal spasm with corkscrew pattern.

The Chicago Classification subtypes of achalasia help predict treatment response. Recent studies showed that type II achalasia patients experience the best treatment response (up to 96%). The lowest response rates were seen in type III achalasia (29–70%) [10]. Opioid use is associated with significantly higher IRP and esophageal manometric patterns consistent with type III achalasia. Therefore caution should be taken during interpretation of these patterns in opioid users [11].

Of note, abnormal EGJ relaxation pressure maybe associated with normal or weak peristalsis that does not meet the criteria for diagnosis of any of the achalasia subtypes. This is suggestive of EGJ outflow obstruction, which can be a manifestation of eosinophilic esophagitis, strictures, LES hypertrophy, paraesophageal hernia, pseudoachalasia or a variant of achalasia [1].

Treatment

While there is no cure for achalasia, current therapies are directed towards reduction of the LES's elevated pressure and improvement of patient's symptoms [4]. Because of their overall ineffectiveness, few studies support oral pharmacologic therapy, e.g. sublingual isosorbide dinitrate or sublingual nifedipine.

Botulinum Toxin Treatment

Botulinum toxin treatment is a safe and easy approach that is capable of LES baseline pressure reduction by about 50% [12]. It disrupts the neurogenic but not the myogenic component of the LES. The standard treatment is injection of 100 units of the toxin in at least four quadrants just above the squamocolumnar junction [4]. Figure 6.3a illustrates this treatment.

While the response rate in the first month can reach up to 75%, the success rate at 1 year is only ~40% requiring repeat injection. It is uncommon to have serious adverse events secondary to this intervention, however up to 25% develop chest pain and on rare occasions mediastinitis occur with inflammatory or allergic reactions. For these reasons use of botulinum toxin treatment should be restricted to patients that are not candidates for endoscopic or surgical therapies.

Endoscopic Pneumatic Dilation

Pneumatic dilation is an effective endoscopic procedure in the management of achalasia. The goal of the procedure is to disrupt the myogenic component of the LES,

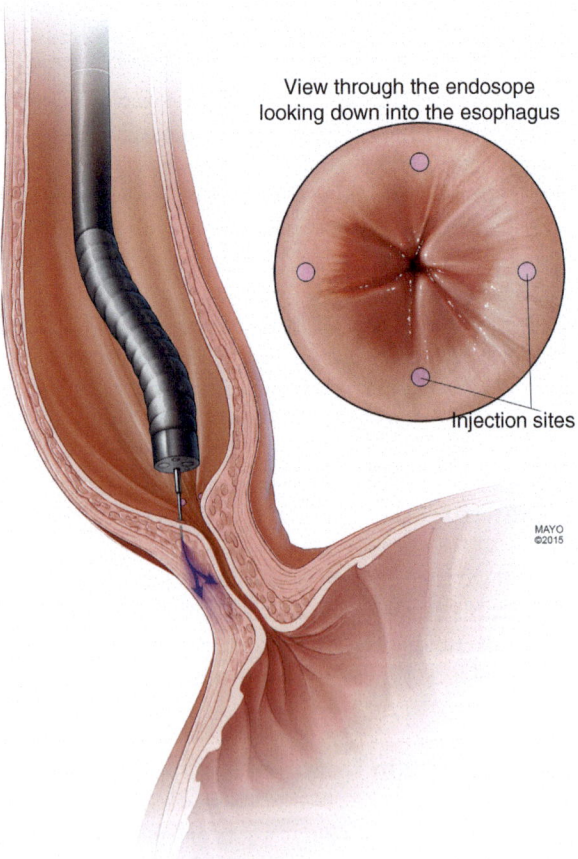

Fig. 6.3 (**a**) Example of botox injection into lower esophageal sphincter. (**b**) Example of pneumatic balloon dilation. (**c**) Example of the Heller myotomy and Toupet and Dor fundoplication

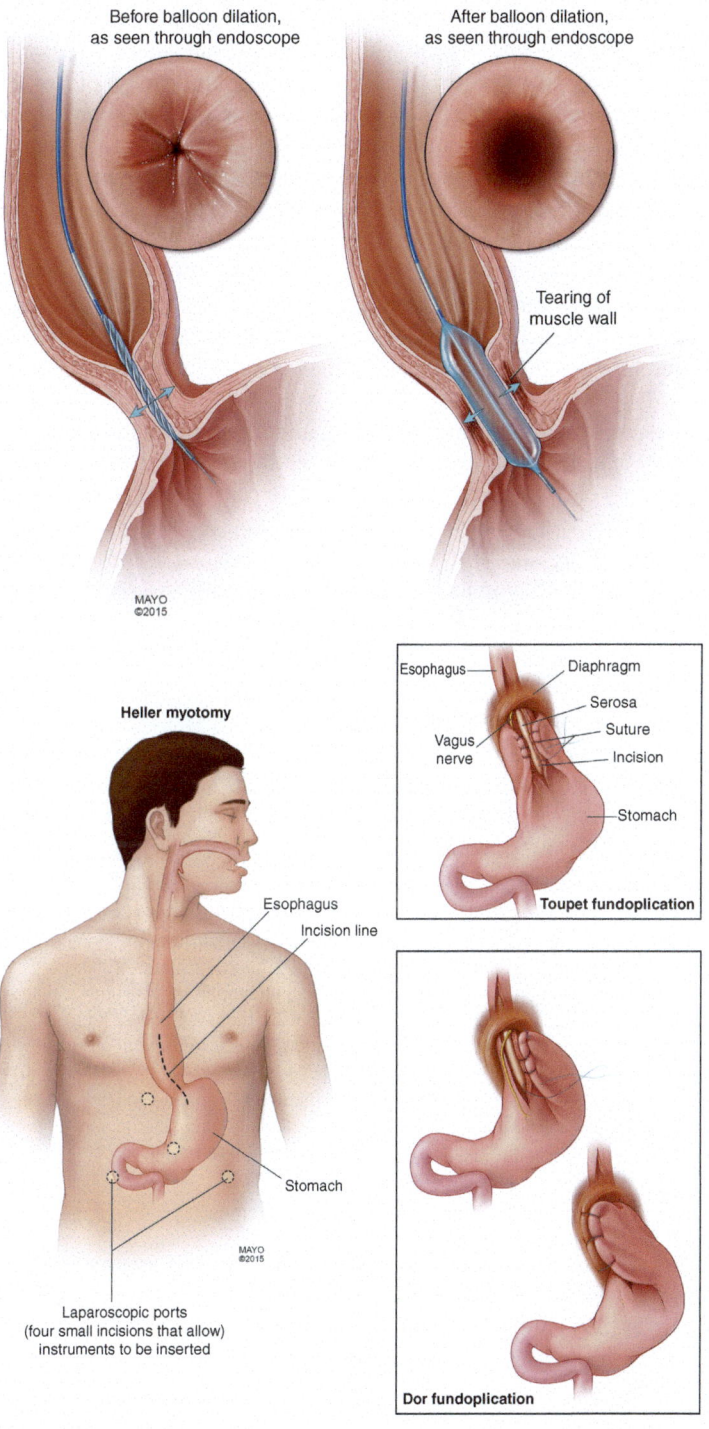

Fig. 6.3 (continued)

i.e. the circular muscle fibers. Air pressure is used to dilate the LES by way of a nonradiopaque polyethylene balloon with fluoroscopy guidance. "Rigiflex dilators" are available in three diameters, 3.0, 3.5 and 4.0 cm. Application of this technique requires expertise in the precise positioning across the LES, as shown in Fig. 6.3b. Distension of the balloon to the maximum diameter is important for effective dilation. The air pressure range is 8–15 psi and is applied between 15 and 60 s [4].

Larger diameter dilations of the LES correlates with increased symptomatic response, such that the greater the size of the dilator (3.0, 3.5 and 4.0 cm) the better symptom relief the patients experience (74, 86 and 90%) over at least the first 1.5 years following dilation [13]. However it has been also shown that more conservative dilations of smaller size (3.0 cm) over a shorter duration (15 s) are equivalent to longer and larger dilations [14]. Serial dilations are superior to single pneumatic dilations [15].

Patient response to treatment with pneumatic dilation is substantial, especially among type II achalasia patients [16]. However about 30% of the patients develop symptom recurrence over the following 5 years. In general, female patients, patients older than 45 years, or those who have a narrow esophagus prior to pneumatic dilation and or an LES pressure < 10 mmHg following dilation are likely to have better treatment response and symptomatic relief. Having type II achalasia on HRM is also predictive of better response to pneumatic dilation. However, male patients younger than 45 years may have suboptimal response to serial dilations. This is likely due to a thicker LES. These patients may benefit from balloons larger than 3.5 cm or may require myomectomy [4, 17].

While pneumatic dilation is a safe outpatient procedure, it may be complicated by esophageal perforation (median rate 1.9%). Therefore radiographic evaluation with gastrograffin should be initiated in the setting of chest pain, vomiting or fever following pneumatic dilation. Small perforation can be managed conservatively with antibiotics, parenteral nutrition and stenting while larger defects may require surgical intervention including thoracotomy. Therefore, patients undergoing pneumatic dilation should be candidates for surgical intervention in case perforation occurs. Lower rates of perforation are seen among those who undergo serial balloon dilations. A more common adverse event of pneumatic dilation is GERD which occur in up to 35% of patients. This may lead to dysphagia secondary to esophageal stricture formation and PPI therapy should be instituted in this setting [4, 15].

Heller Myotomy

Heller myotomy is the standard surgical approach for the treatment of achalasia, which was first described by Ernest Heller in 1913 [18]. It involves division of the circular muscle fibers of the LES, and is successful in up to 94% of patients on long term follow up for up to 36 years. Over the years, minimally invasive laparoscopic myotomy has been developed, providing short term recovery and has lower morbidity rates [4]. Combination of myotomy with fundoplication, also known as modified

Heller myotomy is a more recent excellent surgical strategy with symptomatic relief being achieved in up to 97% of patients [19, 20]. Figure 6.3c illustrates this surgical intervention.

Different myotomy approaches have variable efficacies in terms of symptom improvement. Laparoscopic myotomy (LHM) has the highest efficacy (89%, range 77–100%), followed by the open transabdominal myotomy (85%, range 48–100%) and the thoracoscopic myotomy (78%, range 31–94%) [13]. Long term efficacy of LHM at 6 month and 6 year were 89 and 57%, respectively [4, 15]. Higher response rates are detected among type II achalasia (based on the Chicago Classification v3.0) patients compared to type I and III achalasia. In addition, type III achalasia can be well treated by LHM [16].

Heller myotomy is complicated by GERD in about one third of the cases regardless of the surgical modality, without fundoplication. However combining myotomy with fundoplication decreases the rate of developing GERD to 8–14% [13]. A randomized double-blind controlled trial compared the results on pH studies among those who underwent myotomy with or without fundoplication. It showed that abnormal acid exposure was found in 47% of patients without a fundoplication compared to only 9% among those who had Dor fundoplication performed following myotomy [21]. In addition, this combined technique is more cost effective than myotomy alone given the decreased need for GERD treatment [22]. There is a risk of developing dysphagia among patients undergoing myotomy which is independent from combining it with a fundoplication or not. Nonetheless, PPI therapy is needed for those who complain of heartburn and reflux symptoms after this procedure [4, 13].

Peroral Endoscopic Myotomy

Per-oral endoscopic myotomy (POEM) is an endoscopic approach for the treatment of achalasia. This natural orifice transluminal endoscopic surgery was first described experimentally in 2007 and was first performed in humans in 2008. The initial report showed a significant change in the LES pressure among the pigs who underwent this procedure with a drop from 16.4 to 6.7 mmHg [23, 24]. POEM is safe with excellent efficacy in parallel to surgical myotomy, and is indicated in the treatment of the three achalasia subtypes of Chicago Classification version 3.0 [10, 24, 25].

POEM commonly consists of four endoscopic steps, as shown in Fig. 6.4. Figure 6.4a–f show the procedure in details. Around 2 days prior to POEM, EGD is performed to assess the mucosa and look for food retention. Prophylactic antibiotics are given, commonly a third generation cephalosporin. The initial step in POEM includes a mucosal incision, and then submucosal tunneling followed by myotomy before closure of the mucosal flap. A study of 500 patients who underwent POEM reported a median procedure time of 90 min (interquartile range [IQR] 71–120 min), median myotomy length of 14 cm (IQR 12–16 cm), and median length of hospital stay of 4 days (IQR 4–5 days). The full overview of POEM procedure and its

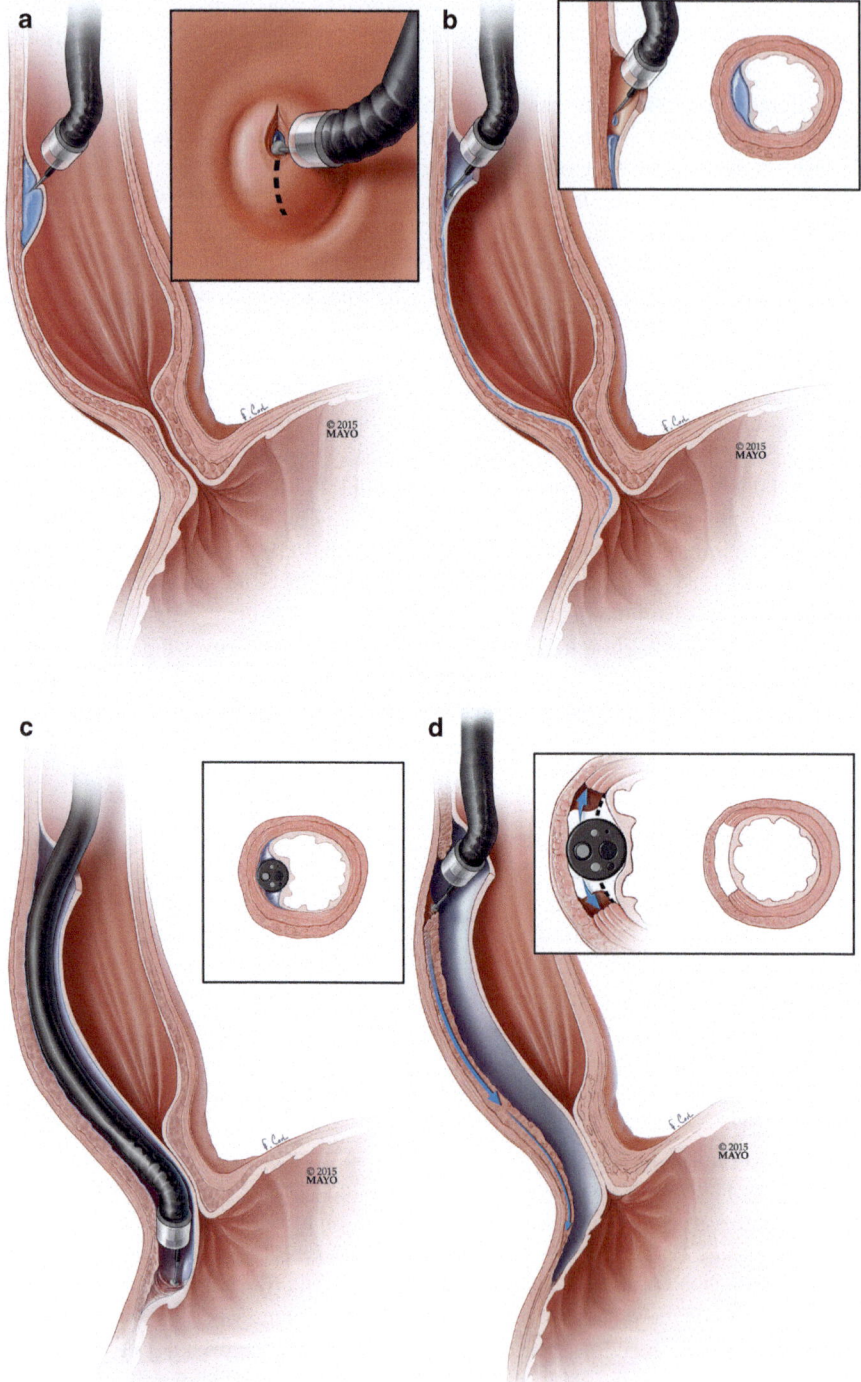

Fig. 6.4 POEM procedure. Figures (**a**)–(**f**) show the procedure in details

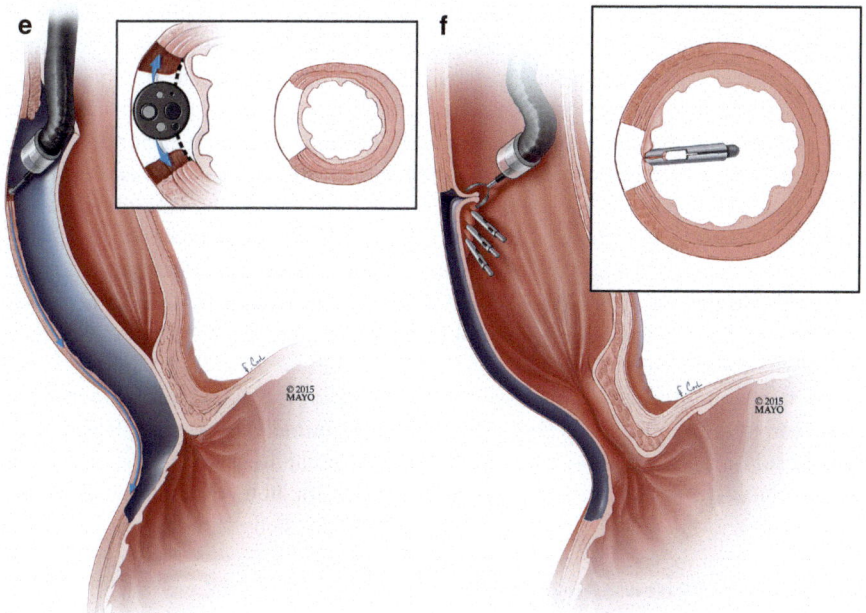

Fig. 6.4 (continued)

technical details can be reviewed at the American Society of Gastrointestinal Endoscopy website (*www.giejournal.org*) (video of the procedure is also available) [24, 25].

Success of the procedure can be assessed using a timed barium esophagram and measuring a change in LES pressure and IRP as well as the GEJ distensibility index. Clinically the Eckardt score can assess for symptom improvement, with a score of <3 suggesting a successful outcome. Inoue et al. showed a decrease in the Eckardt score from 6 (range 5–8) before POEM to 1 (range 1–2) at 3 years ($p < 0.01$). In the same study, the decrease in the median LES pressure was from 25 mm Hg (range 18–35 mm Hg) to 12 (range 10–15 mm Hg) at 3 years. Such findings were supported by international prospective multicenter studies and meta-analyses. In addition, the quality of life of patients with achalasia who underwent POEM improved significantly. This was assessed using the short form SF-36 [24, 25].

Efficacy of POEM has been evaluated by the American Society for Gastrointestinal Endoscopy PIVI (Preservation and Incorporation of Valuable Endoscopic Innovations). The threshold efficacy was set at 80% at least 12 months after the procedure. This was defined as Eckardt score ≤3 (dysphagia component of ≤2) and a ≤6% serious adverse event rate. The 30-day mortality rate was ≤0.1% [26]. While efficacy of other treatment approaches (LHM and PD) is low in type III achalasia, POEM is effective in type III achalasia of Chicago Classification with symptom relief in 91% of patients at 24-month follow up [10, 27]. In octogenarians POEM is also safe and efficacious with up to 91% success rate on median follow up of 8–9 months [28].

Some studies reported persistence of GERD symptoms in less than one third of the patients. Adverse events has been reported with variable rates and include: endoscopic evidence of esophageal erosions, pneumo–/capnoperitoneum, pneumo–/capnomediastinum, pneumo–/capnothorax, aspiration pneumonia, subcutaneous emphysema, mucosal flap injury, accidental full-thickness muscle perforation, peritonitis, mucosal ulceration, submucosal hematoma, pleural effusions and atelectasis, leaks and perforations, esophageal strictures, dehiscence at tunnel entry, submucosal fistula, seizures and atrial fibrillation [26]. In octogenarians, a study of 76 patients with mean age of 84 years showed that in patients with achalasia (type I-III) who underwent POEM procedure, adverse events were slightly higher than in previous reports. Six capnoperitoneum/mediastinum were symptomatic and there were two esophageal leaks [28].

Certain comorbidities including cirrhosis with portal hypertension and prior radiotherapy of the thorax or abdomen may be contraindications to POEM. It may also be contraindicated in patients with prior endoscopic interventions of the esophagus including mucosal ablation, mucosal resection or submucosal dissection [24].

Controversies in Management

Achalasia subtypes of the Chicago Classification help predict treatment response. Type II achalasia patients experience the best treatment response (up to 96%), however type III achalasia is associated with the lowest response rates (29–70%) [10]. Type I & II achalasia respond to either endoscopic or surgical therapies (LHM, Pneumatic dilation, and POEM). Achalasia type III responds best to POEM [20, 27, 29]. Botulinum toxin treatment should be reserved for patients who are poor candidates for endoscopic or surgical therapies. Except for select patients where PD is a potential treatment option, POEM and LHM with fundoplication remains the main treatment modality for achalasia. Standard myotomy of the LES should be adequate in classic achalasia (achalasia types I and II), while extensive myotomy is preferred in type III achalasia to achieve a better clinical response. Extensive myotomy can be achieved with POEM [30].

POEM has favorable outcomes when compared with other treatment modalities. A randomized controlled multicenter trial (RCT) in 133 treatment naïve patients with achalasia showed that POEM had higher success rates compared to PD, 92 vs. 70% respectively. One esophageal perforation was reported as a major adverse event in the PD group. No major adverse events were reported among patients who underwent POEM. GERD was reported following POEM among 49% of patients based on pH monitoring compared to 39% of patients who underwent PD and 9% who underwent LHM with fundoplication [13, 26]. POEM was associated with higher clinical success rates compared to LHM with fundoplication for achalasia type III. The reported response rates were 98% in the POEM group compared to 80% in the LHM with fundoplication group. This is due to POEM's ability to perform an extensive myotomy (16 vs. 8 cm). Comparison of both groups showed that POEM was associated with shorter procedure time and lower rates of adverse events (6 vs. 27%). However, patients who underwent POEM had a shorter follow up period (8.6 vs. 21.5 months) [30].

In experienced centers, POEM was associated with 0–1% major adverse events and 92–100% success rates despite having a short term follow up. Post POEM GERD occurred at a rate of 22–53%, and 0–3% required additional anti-reflux surgery. The endoscopic modality of POEM does not allow performance of anti-reflux surgery. However anti-reflux surgery may not be necessary in all patients undergoing POEM. Similarly fundoplication is not absolutely necessary following LHM. With limited hiatal dissection, LHM with or without Dor fundoplication was associated with similar rates of GERD at 3 year followup [31]. Recently, endoscopic anti reflux mucosectomy (ARM) procedure was described for post POEM GERD. Surgical fundoplication is an option if ARM fail, especially if the patient has a significant hiatal hernia [32].

The POEM procedure has gained acceptance worldwide in less than a decade. It changed the treatment paradigm of achalasia. However, further research studies are needed to further evaluate the technical aspect of this procedure and its' outcomes. This include full thickness versus circular muscle myotomy, anterior versus posterior approach of POEM, endoscopist positioning, type of knife, injectant for the tunnel, fluoroscopy-assisted determination of the GE junction and endoscopic closure methods (clipping vs. suturing). The learning curve of POEM is a limitation [24].

POEM is a safe and effective treatment modality for achalasia. In experienced centers, it is not limited by age, esophageal anatomy (even in sigmoid esophagus), or history of prior treatment for achalasia. Adverse event rates are low and are rarely clinically significant. If POEM procedure fails, repeat POEM has been successful in most cases. Esophagectomy may be considered if LHM has failed. Treatment for achalasia should be tailored based on patient characteristics, patient preference and local expertise until prospective randomized controlled trials with long term follow up are available.

References

1. Vaezi MF, Richter JE. Diagnosis and management of achalasia. American College of Gastroenterology Practice Parameter Committee. Am J Gastroenterol. 1999;94(12):3406–12.
2. Francis DL, Katzka DA. Achalasia: update on the disease and its treatment. Gastroenterology. 2010;139(2):369–74.
3. Pandolfino JE, Kahrilas PJ. Presentation, diagnosis, and management of achalasia. Clin Gastroenterol Hepatol. 2013;11(8):887–97.
4. Vaezi MF, Pandolfino JE, Vela MF. ACG clinical guideline: diagnosis and management of achalasia. Am J Gastroenterol. 2013;108(8):1238–49; quiz 1250
5. Andersson M, et al. Evaluation of the response to treatment in patients with idiopathic achalasia by the timed barium esophagogram: results from a randomized clinical trial. Dis Esophagus. 2009;22(3):264–73.
6. Kahrilas PJ, et al. Comparison of pseudoachalasia and achalasia. Am J Med. 1987;82(3):439–46.
7. Savarino E, et al. Achalasia with dense eosinophilic infiltrate responds to steroid therapy. Clin Gastroenterol Hepatol. 2011;9(12):1104–6.
8. Pandolfino JE, et al. High-resolution manometry in clinical practice: utilizing pressure topography to classify oesophageal motility abnormalities. Neurogastroenterol Motil. 2009;21(8):796–806.
9. Kahrilas PJ, et al. The Chicago classification of esophageal motility disorders, v3.0. Neurogastroenterol Motil. 2015;27(2):160–74.

10. Rohof WOA, Bredenoord AJ. Chicago classification of esophageal motility disorders: lessons learned. Curr Gastroenterol Rep. 2017;19(8):37.
11. Ratuapli SK, et al. Opioid-induced esophageal dysfunction (OIED) in patients on chronic opioids. Am J Gastroenterol. 2015;110(7):979–84.
12. Hoogerwerf WA, Pasricha PJ. Pharmacologic therapy in treating achalasia. Gastrointest Endosc Clin N Am. 2001;11(2):311–24, vii.
13. Campos GM, et al. Endoscopic and surgical treatments for achalasia: a systematic review and meta-analysis. Ann Surg. 2009;249(1):45–57.
14. Gideon RM, Castell DO, Yarze J. Prospective randomized comparison of pneumatic dilatation technique in patients with idiopathic achalasia. Dig Dis Sci. 1999;44(9):1853–7.
15. Vela MF, et al. The long-term efficacy of pneumatic dilatation and Heller myotomy for the treatment of achalasia. Clin Gastroenterol Hepatol. 2006;4(5):580–7.
16. Rohof WO, et al. Outcomes of treatment for achalasia depend on manometric subtype. Gastroenterology. 2013;144(4):718–25; quiz e13-4
17. Pratap N, et al. Achalasia cardia subtyping by high-resolution manometry predicts the therapeutic outcome of pneumatic balloon dilatation. J Neurogastroenterol Motil. 2011;17(1):48–53.
18. Payne WS. Heller's contribution to the surgical treatment of achalasia of the esophagus. 1914. Ann Thorac Surg. 1989;48(6):876–81.
19. Litle VR. Laparoscopic Heller myotomy for achalasia: a review of the controversies. Ann Thorac Surg. 2008;85(2):S743–6.
20. Zaninotto G, et al. Four hundred laparoscopic myotomies for esophageal achalasia: a single centre experience. Ann Surg. 2008;248(6):986–93.
21. Richards WO, et al. Heller myotomy versus Heller myotomy with Dor fundoplication for achalasia: a prospective randomized double-blind clinical trial. Ann Surg. 2004;240(3):405–12; discussion 412-5
22. Torquati A, et al. Laparoscopic myotomy for achalasia: predictors of successful outcome after 200 cases. Ann Surg. 2006;243(5):587–91; discussion 591-3
23. Pasricha PJ, et al. Submucosal endoscopic esophageal myotomy: a novel experimental approach for the treatment of achalasia. Endoscopy. 2007;39(9):761–4.
24. Pannala R, et al. Per-oral endoscopic myotomy (with video). Gastrointest Endosc. 2016;83(6):1051–60.
25. Inoue H, et al. Per-oral endoscopic myotomy: a series of 500 patients. J Am Coll Surg. 2015;221(2):256–64.
26. American Society for Gastrointestinal Endoscopy, P.C, et al. The American Society for Gastrointestinal Endoscopy PIVI (Preservation and Incorporation of Valuable Endoscopic Innovations) on peroral endoscopic myotomy. Gastrointest Endosc. 2015;81(5):1087–100 e1.
27. Zhang W, Linghu EQ. Peroral endoscopic myotomy for type III achalasia of Chicago classification: outcomes with a minimum follow-up of 24 months. J Gastrointest Surg. 2017;21(5):785–91.
28. Chen YI, et al. An international multicenter study evaluating the clinical efficacy and safety of per-oral endoscopic myotomy in octogenarians. Gastrointest Endosc. 2017. https://doi.org/10.1016/j.gie.2017.02.007.
29. Kahrilas PJ, Pandolfino JE. Treatments for achalasia in 2017: how to choose among them. Curr Opin Gastroenterol. 2017;33(4):270–6.
30. Kumbhari V, et al. Peroral endoscopic myotomy (POEM) vs laparoscopic Heller myotomy (LHM) for the treatment of type III achalasia in 75 patients: a multicenter comparative study. Endosc Int Open. 2015;3(3):E195–201.
31. Simic AP, et al. Significance of limited hiatal dissection in surgery for achalasia. J Gastrointest Surg. 2010;14(4):587–93.
32. Bechara R, Inoue H. Recent advancement of therapeutic endoscopy in the esophageal benign diseases. World J Gastrointest Endosc. 2015;7(5):481–95.

Paraesophageal Hernia

7

Gurteshwar Rana, Priscila Rodrigues Armijo,
Crystal Krause, and Dmitry Oleynikov

Introduction

Herniation through the esophageal hiatus was not well-described prior to the advent of the x-ray. Hiatal hernias were first described in detail by Henry Ingersoll Bowditch in Boston in 1853, and were first classified into three primary subtypes by the Swedish radiologist, Ake Akerlund, in 1926 [1]. Hiatal hernias are defined as a prolapse of a portion of the stomach through the diaphragmatic esophageal hiatus [2]. These diaphragmatic defects may be related to an increase in intraabdominal pressure, leading to a trans-diaphragmatic pressure gradient between the thoracic and abdominal cavities at the gastroesophageal junction (GEJ) [3]. This pressure gradient may lead to widening of the diaphragmatic hiatus through a weakening of the phrenoesophageal membrane. A variety of conditions can contribute to the increase in intraabdominal pressure, including obesity, pregnancy, chronic constipation, and chronic obstructive pulmonary disease with chronic cough. Both acquired and genetic factors may contributed to the development of hiatal hernias, as some studies have shown that there are specific familial clusters of hernia development across

G. Rana
Department of Surgery, University of Nebraska Medical Center, 986245 Nebraska Medical Center, Omaha, NE, USA

P. R. Armijo · C. Krause
Center for Advanced Surgical Technology, University of Nebraska Medical Center, 986245 Nebraska Medical Center, Omaha, NE, USA

D. Oleynikov, M.D., F.A.C.S. (✉)
Department of Surgery, University of Nebraska Medical Center, 986245 Nebraska Medical Center, Omaha, NE, USA

Center for Advanced Surgical Technology, University of Nebraska Medical Center, 986245 Nebraska Medical Center, Omaha, NE, USA
e-mail: doleynik@unmc.edu

© Springer International Publishing AG, part of Springer Nature 2018
D. Oleynikov, P. M. Fisichella (eds.), *A Mastery Approach to Complex Esophageal Diseases*, https://doi.org/10.1007/978-3-319-75795-7_7

generations, indicating a possible autosomal dominant mode of inheritance. Some evidence has linked a collagen-encoding COL3A1 gene and an altered collagen-remodeling mechanism in the formation of hiatal hernias [4, 5].

Hiatal hernias were originally classified into three types, but the current classification scheme defines four types of hiatal or paraesophageal hernias, based on the contents of the hernia sac [5, 6]. Type 1, also referred to as a "sliding hernia", is characterized by an increased diameter of the hiatal passage and decrease in circumferential strength of the phrenoesophageal membrane, resulting in the migration of the GEJ into the thorax. The Type 2 hernia results from the herniation of the gastric fundus through a weakness in the phrenoesophageal membrane, but the GEJ remains in the normal anatomic location. This type of hernia is sometimes referred to as a "true PEH or rolling hernia". The Type 3 hernias, sometimes termed "giant PEHs", can consist of a combination of Types 1 and 2, involving a herniation of the GEJ and stomach into the thoracic cavity. Type 4 hernias consist of other intraabdominal viscera, such as colon, small bowel, omentum, or spleen along with the stomach in the hernia sac. Type 1 hiatal hernias are the most common, and account for nearly 95% of all hiatal hernias, with the other three types combining to make the remaining 5% [6]. When patients are symptomatic, all of these types of hernias can be approached with similar preoperative and operative strategies.

Clinical Presentation and Diagnostic Procedures

While the true prevalence of these hernias is difficult to determine because they are often asymptomatic or poorly defined, more recent epidemiologic studies have shown them to be more common than previously recognized in the Western population [4]. A typical PEH patient is female, commonly in or beyond their sixth decade of life, and may present with vague symptoms of intermittent epigastric pain and postprandial fullness. Type 1 or sliding hernias are commonly associated with gastroesophageal reflux disease (GERD). Large hiatal defects (such as those present in Type 3 and 4), often present with symptoms of progressive intolerance to solids/liquids with regurgitation, nausea, and vomiting. The symptoms that present are often related to the space that the hernia occupies in the thoracic cavity, such as chest pain and respiratory problems due to lung compression or aspiration. These respiratory issues may include shortness of breath, asthma, and bronchitis. Other unpredictable symptoms which may be revealed with a thorough history include hoarseness, cough, laryngitis, and pharyngitis [4]. Cameron lesions related to hiatal hernias can be an unusual cause of gastrointestinal bleeding and iron deficiency anemia. These lesions are characterized by linear gastric ulcers or erosions located on the gastric mucosal folds at the diaphragmatic impression of large hiatal hernias [7]. Cameron lesions are prevalent in 5% of patients with a hiatal hernia discovered on upper endoscopy, and the risk of one existing increases with hernia size [7]. More acute complications of PEHs are mechanical problems such as gastric obstruction, volvulus, incarceration and strangulation which require urgent surgical intervention. These problems may be seen in a patient who presents with obstructive symptoms of new onset dysphagia, chest pain, and early satiety. There is a well-known triad, Borchardt's triad, associated with gastric volvulus that one should look for in patients: epigastric pain, inability to vomit, and failure to pass a nasogastric tube into the stomach [8]. Some long-term effects of hiatal hernias are the development of severe reflux with associated erosive esophagitis, Barrett's esophagus, and an increased risk of subsequent esophageal cancer [4]. All symptomatic patients are recommended to undergo PEH repair if deemed to be a good surgical candidate.

Preoperative Evaluation

Hiatal hernias may be revealed during the work-up of unexplained upper gastrointestinal (GI) symptoms, cardiac, or respiratory symptoms, or can be discovered incidentally on lateral chest radiographs as a retro-cardiac bubble. The evaluation of these patients should follow a standard protocol in all instances, including a complete history and physical. The history may reveal symptoms that were not previously apparent. The physical examination of these patients is usually unremarkable unless they are having acute complications related to the hiatal hernia. The best diagnostic study to determine the presence and size of the hernia is an upper GI barium study. It can also demonstrate associated esophageal motility dysfunction or stricture/stenosis related to long-standing GERD [4]. Esophagogastroduodenoscopy (EGD) is essential to evaluating esophageal length and the mucosa of the herniated stomach for any other abnormal pathology such as ulcers, esophagitis, gastritis, Barrett's esophagus, or neoplasms. EGDs should be performed on all patients who are being evaluated for PEH repair in order to better understand the important anatomic landmarks specific to each patient. Esophageal manometry is also essential to assess esophageal motility and lower esophageal sphincter characteristics (pressure, relaxation, and location) which may alter the operative approach with regards to the choice of fundoplication performed. Though not essential in the preoperative evaluation, an esophageal pH study can help to provide a quantitative analysis of reflux episodes by correlating pH with a patient's subjective complaints of reflux [3]. Often, because these patients are elderly, they have significant comorbidities that require further evaluation, specifically with regard to assessment of cardiac and respiratory status. With the help of anesthesia, cardiology, and pulmonology preoperative consultations, the necessary additional studies (such as cardiac stress tests or pulmonary function tests) are obtained. All of these examinations help to determine whether or not the patient is a suitable surgical candidate.

Treatment

The majority of patients who are symptomatic will experience little relief for their upper GI symptoms with over-the-counter antacids, histamine (H2) receptor antagonists, or proton pump inhibitors (PPIs). These medications may assist in controlling the symptoms of the hiatal hernia, and it may be useful to continue these medications, the definitive management of PEHs is surgery. PEHs have been tradi- tionally treated with a thoracotomy or laparotomy, but the transabdominal laparo- scopic approach is increasing accepted as the preferred approach for the repair of hiatal hernias. Laparoscopic PEH repair was first reported in 1991 and this approach has continued to evolve with respect to variations in technique, including removal or reduction of the hernia sac, the use of mesh to reinforce the cruroplasty, and whether or not to incorporate an anti-reflux procedure. Despite these controversies in practice, certain basic tenants exist in laparoscopic hiatal hernia repair: reduction of the hernia sac and its contents, complete dissection of both crura and the GEJ, tension free re-approximation of the hiatus, and adequate mobilization of the esoph- agus to achieve at least 3 cm of intra-abdominal esophagus [3].

Laparoscopic Paraesophageal Hernia Repair Procedure

We perform the laparoscopic PEH procedure with the patient in steep reverse Trendelenburg position, with a footboard at the base of the bed and a belt strap at the waist. Both arms are tucked and padded appropriately to minimize neurologic injury. Since the procedure can take some time, a Foley catheter is placed for accu- rate measurement of urine output, and an orogastric tube is inserted for stomach decompression. The patient will have received preoperative antibiotics and chemi- cal and mechanical venous thromboembolism prophylaxis. A video monitor is at the head of the bed so that both operators are able to view the screen.

Figure 7.1 shows the arrangement of laparoscopic ports for the appropriate trian- gulation of working space in the hiatus. After insufflation, the esophageal hiatus will be slightly to the patient's left, and both the mediastinum and the esophageal hiatus will be more cephalad. Care must be taken to ensure that the laparoscopic ports are placed high enough and slightly to the left on the patient's abdominal wall. For the trocar placement, a 2 mm incision is made in the left upper quadrant (LUQ)

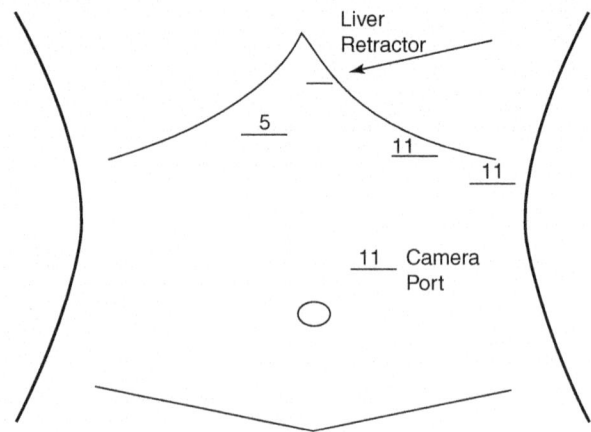

Fig. 7.1 Port placement

and then a Veress needle is used to access the abdomen. After the Veress needle is confirmed by saline drop test to be intra-abdominal, pneumoperitoneum is achieved by insufflation of the abdomen with CO_2 at 15 mm Hg.

An 11 mm visualization trocare is placed approximately 10 cm superior and 2 cm lateral to umbilicus (to the patient's left). Three additional working ports are added (11 mm in LUQ, 11 mm more lateral on the left, and a 5 mm in RUQ which will go through the falciform ligament), and a Nathanson liver retractor is added through a 5 mm epigastric incision (Fig. 7.1).

After the ports are added, the complete reduction of the hernia sac can begin. The patient is put in steep reverse Trendelenburg and a right-side-down position to optimize view of the hiatus. The contents of the hernia sac are pulled down below the diaphragm. Figure 7.2 shows a large Type 3 PEH. Starting with a left crus approach at the level of the inferior splenic pole, a bipolar energy device is used to divide the short gastrics. The left crus is dissected at the angle of His and the mediastinal space is entered in the avascular plane directly anterior to the aorta (Fig. 7.3). Continue the

Fig. 7.2 Large Type 3 paraesophageal hernia

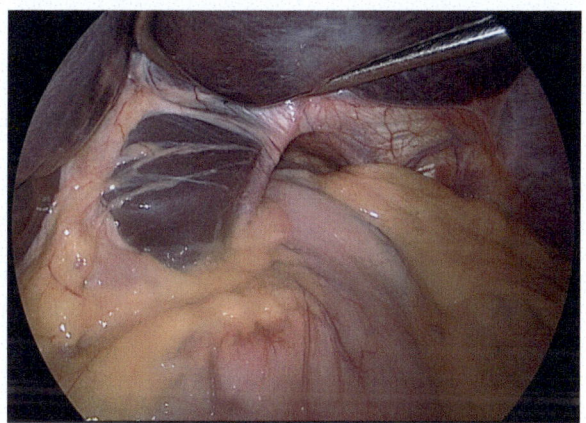

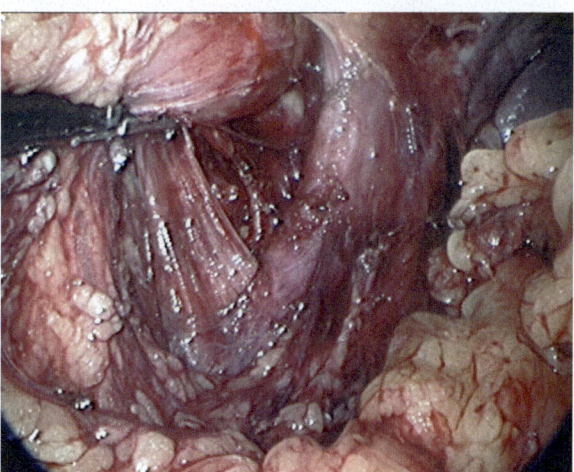

Fig. 7.3 Dissection of left crus

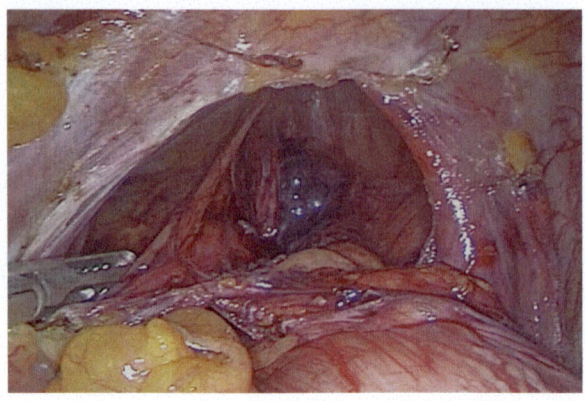

Fig. 7.4 Anterior
dissection

circumferential dissection anterior to the esophagus until the medial edge of the
right crus can be visualized (Fig. 7.4). At this point, switch to the dissection of the
alternate side, using the bipolar energy device to divide the gastrohepatic ligament.
Starting at the decussation and moving anteriorly, continue the dissection just
medial to the right crus, always being aware of the location of the posterior vagus
nerve. After creation of a retoresophageal window, a Penrose drain is inserted into
the posterior plane to increase the esophageal traction by the surgical assistant.

Extensive mediastinal dissection is needed in order to obtain the necessary 3 cm
of intra-abdominal esophagus. This step is important for achieving an appropriate
esophageal length to avoid the need to perform a Collis gastroplasty and the subsequent complications that are associated with this procedure. The mediastinal dissection can be aided by the removal of the orogastric tube, which allows for increased
esophageal retraction (Fig. 7.5). The use of the electrocautery hook is useful for
dissection in this area, as vascular attachments are often present.

For the creation of a tension-free posterior cruroplasty with mesh reinforcement,
place a series of interrupted sutures posterior to the esophagus every 5–8 mm. This
will ensure adequate bites of tissue on both crura. For the final two sutures, decrease
the pneumoperitoneum to approximately 8 mm Hg in order to decrease the tension
on the diaphragm (Fig. 7.6). The absorbable mesh is secured to the left and right
crus, posteriorly in a U-shaped overlay fashion to support the cruroplasty (Fig. 7.7).

Based on the results of the preoperative esophageal manometry test, a standard
Nissen or Toupet fundoplication is performed. If inadequate esophageal motility is
observed, a Toupet fundoplication will be used in order to minimize the potential for
postoperative dysphagia. To begin the fundoplication, a location on the greater curvature of the stomach that is 3 cm distal and posterior to the GEJ is marked with a
clip. The standard "shoeshine" maneuver is used in order to creat a floppy, sym-
metrical fundoplication. The wrap is secured with interrupted sutures, approximately 2 cm apart, either to the opposing side of the stomach or to the esophagus
depending on whether it is a Nissen or Toupet, respectively. The Penrose drain is
removed after the first suture, and the fundoplication s secured to the hiatus via
stitches on both crura, taking bites of the wrap, esophagus, and diaphragm (Fig. 7.8).

Fig. 7.5 Complete reduction of hernia sac and esophageal mobilization

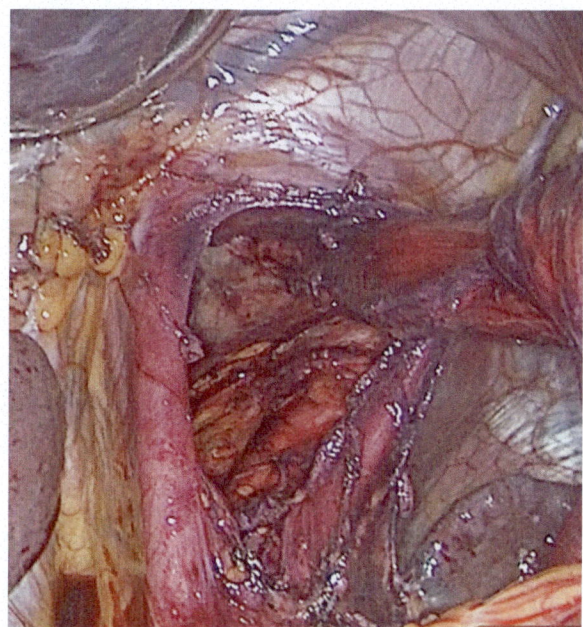

Fig. 7.6 Posterior cruroplasty

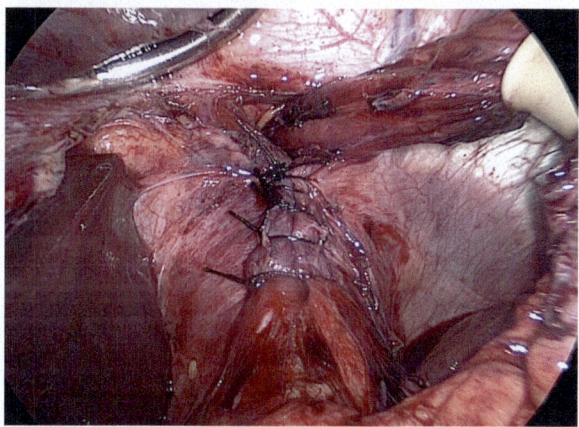

At the completion of the procedure, a routine endoscopy is performed in order to confirm smoot entry into the stomach at the GEJ and to visualize the completed wrap to ensure symmetry on retroflexion (Fig. 7.9).

The patient is started on a clear liquid diet on postoperative day 0 and advanced the next day to a soft mechanical diet. An upper GI is not routinely performed postoperatively, and patients are usually discharged home on postoperative day 1. Patients are instructed to continue a diet of soft food for the first 2 weeks until their first postoperative visit in the clinic. All patients are routinely seen again in clinic at 6 months and 12 months post-procedure.

Fig. 7.7 Mesh insertion
and retraction of esophagus
with Penrose drain

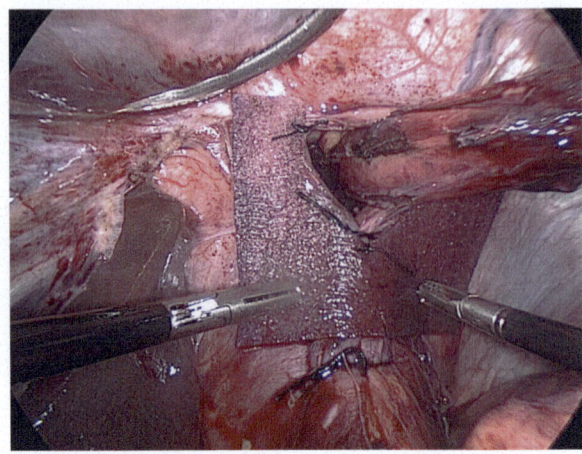

Fig. 7.8 Toupet
fundoplication

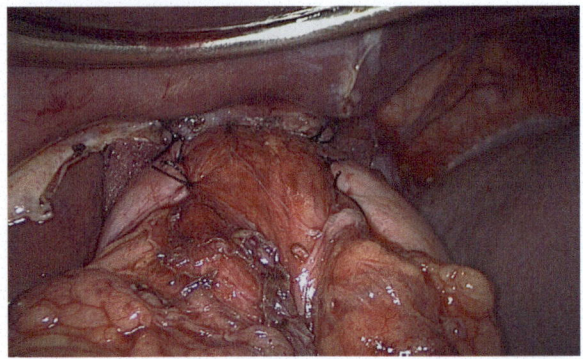

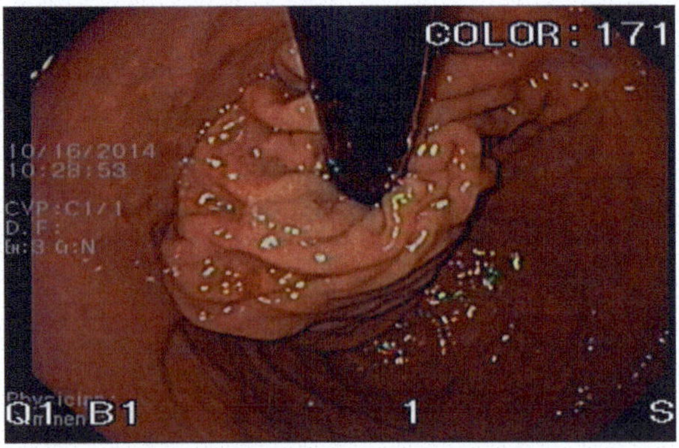

Fig. 7.9 Completion
endoscopy showing
symmetric Nissen
fundoplication

Key Technical Points in Laparoscopic PEH Repair
1. Complete reduction of the hernia sac after careful dissection.
2. Identification of the GEJ and both crura.
3. Obtaining adequate intra-abdominal esophageal length, at least 3 cm.
4. Tension-free re-approximation of the crura, utilizing onlay mesh.
5. Creation of an anti-reflux procedure to help restore lower esophageal sphincter competency and secure the repair.
6. Completion endoscopy to ensure proper fundoplication technique.

Controversies in Technique

Laparoscopic hernia repair has been proven to be a safe a feasible procedure, with improved outcomes when compared to its open counterpart, and the majority of surgeons now accept it as the standard of care. For the patients, the laparoscopic approach provides fast recovery, shorter hospital stays, reduced pulmonary complications, faster recovery, and less morbidity. Surgeons take advantage of the better visualization during the mediastinal dissection allowing for greater esophageal lengthening and decreased need to perform a Collis gastroplasty [9, 10]. A literature view by Draaisma et al. found that patients undergoing laparoscopic hiatal hernia repair had an overall median hospital stay of 3 days, and a morbidity rate of 4.3% [11]. Those rates were significantly higher for the conventional open patients, who had an overall mean length of stay of 10 days, and a morbidity rate of 16.2% [11]. Though not demonstrated in all studies, one area in which the laparoscopic PEH repair has been shown to be less superior than the open repair is in recurrence rates [12]. Thus, modifications have been made to the technical aspects of this surgery in order to lower the recurrence rates, some of which are controversial. These controversial techniques include topics such as complete removal of the hernia sac, the need to perform an anti-reflux procedure, placement of a gastrostomy tube or gastropexy, or the use of mesh (and which type is best) to reinforce the cruroplasty [12, 13].

The performance of an anti-reflux procedure with laparoscopic PEH repair is the standard of care in several institutions throughout the United States, such as the University of Nebraska Medical Center. This technique not only helps to prevent recurrence, but also aids in re-establishing the lower esophageal sphincter (LES) pressure [12]. The addition of fundoplication in PEH can relieve or resolve the symptoms of reflux in the majority of patients with paraesophageal hernias who present with those symptoms prior to the repair. Based on preoperative 24-hour pH studies and manometry, 60–100% of these patients will have GERD and/or decreased lower esophageal sphincter pressure [8]. In addition, the fundoplication helps to restore the disruption of the normal anatomy of the LES that occurs during the trans-hiatal dissection, treating the subsequent postoperative reflux. In 2011, a prospective study compared patients who received a fundoplication to those who underwent a cruroplasty [14]. The group with no fundoplication had an increased incidence of new-onset esophagitis of 28 vs. 7% in patients who received a fundoplication. It also showed an increase in the number of abnormal pH tests postoperatively in the group without a fundoplication, from 29% preoperatively to 44% after surgery [14]. Besides combatting postoperative reflux, the fundoplication may act as an anchor to keep the stomach below the diaphragm and reduce hernia recurrence. Whether performing a Nissen or a 270° fundoplication can be assessed by preoperative manometry studies, which help to determine which will be best suited for the patient. A Toupet fundoplication is usually indicated for patients with esophageal dysmotility disorders [15]. Many studies have published lower dysphagia rates after Toupet fundoplication compared with Nissen with little difference in control of GERD after 1–5 years of follow-up [16]. An anti-reflux procedure, whether a Nissen or a Toupet, is key to restoring the mechanical barrier to reflux and should be part of all laparoscopic paraesophageal hernia repairs.

The use of mesh is another area of PEH repair that has often come under debate. Certain comparative studies have shown that patients with a prosthetic hiatal closure have a lower rate of postoperative hiatal hernia recurrence in comparison to patients with simple hiatal repair in laparoscopic PEH repair operations [17]. There are concerns, however, with using a prosthetic mesh because of associated complications such as adhesion formation, mesh contraction, foreign body reaction, and tissue erosion that may lead to revisional surgery [18]. Another problem associated with mesh hiatoplasty is the increased frequency of patients complaining of late dysphagia with a prevalence of up to 13% [19]. A review of 28 cases of mesh-related complications by Stadlhuber et al. demonstrated reoperative findings of intraluminal mesh erosion ($n = 17$), esophageal stenosis ($n = 6$), and dense fibrosis ($n = 5$) [20]. There was no relationship in this study to any particular mesh as these complications occurred in patients who had undergone hiatal hernia repair with polypropylene, polytetrafluoroethylene (PTFE), biologic, or dual mesh and subsequently presented with symptoms of dysphagia, heartburn, chest pain, fever, epigastric pain, and weight loss [20]. The choice to use absorbable mesh in the place of synthetic meshes is to minimize some of these morbidities. In the literature review by Antoniou et al., porcine dermal collagen (PDC) mesh was shown by several studies to have decreased adhesion formation and fibrosis and enhanced neovascularization which demonstrate the advantages of biologic implants over synthetic meshes [19]. Oelschlager and colleagues investigated the use of porcine small intestinal submucosa as a biologic mesh to supplement laparoscopic PEH repair in a multicenter, prospective trial consisting of 108 patients who were randomized to repair with or without this onlay, keyhole-shaped biologic mesh. After 6 months, 90% of the study group underwent UGI testing, and results indicated a significant reduction in recurrence rates in the mesh patient population versus the nonmesh group (9% compared to 24%, respectively) without any mesh-related complications [19, 21]. One study by Schmidt and colleagues compared mesh repair (onlay biologic) versus primary suture repair among 70 patients with small hiatal defects less than 5 cm. At 1 year after surgery, the patients were studied with a barium swallow and/or EGD to assess for recurrence. For the suture cruroplasty group, 5 of 32 patients (16%) demonstrated recurrence while none of the 38 patients which had crural reinforcement with absorbable mesh recurred ($p = 0.017$) [22]. Lee et al. studied the results of using human acellular dermal matrix mesh in laparoscopic hiatal hernia repair in 52 patients after 1 year and demonstrated a recurrence rate of only 3.8% and no mesh-related complications [23]. An absorbable mesh cruroplasty helps to decrease the early recurrence rate of PEHs after laparoscopic repair without increasing the complication rate. Further studies are necessary to help determine the long-term recurrence rates and their significance after laparoscopic PEH repair with absorbable mesh.

Gastropexy is an alternative to PEH repair without mesh. However, few studies have evaluated its outcomes, and no randomized trials exist. The anterior gastropexy was first described by Boerema in 1958 [13]. However, high long-term recurrence rates lead to a modified technique with the addition of fundoplication [13]. One study analyzed 89 patients who had underwent laparoscopic repair of a large PEH without mesh, but with fundoplication and anterior gastropexy. These patients had a recurrence rate of 15.7%, with good functional results in 75.3% of patients after a mean follow-up of 57.5 months [24]. However, since no data was available concerning long-term barium swallow studies, the recurrence rates could have been higher if the study had included patients with asymptomatic radiologic recurrence [19]. A multicenter, prospective study of 101 patients who underwent PEH repair using a modified Boerema technique without fundoplication found a similar recurrence rate of 16.8%. The authors reported that almost 30% of patients had postoperative reflux, with 10% requiring daily PPI. This study also had limitations, including a lower than expected incidence of reported recurrence, potentially due to either a short follow-up time (average of 10 months), or underreported radiographic recurrence [13]. A most recent case report in Japan found that laparoscopic PEH repair with anterior gastropexy can be a safe and feasible alternative in elderly patients with multiple comorbidities [25]. Still, further studies, including clinical randomized trials, are required to fully understand the role of anterior gastropexy in the repair of paraesophageal hernia.

Conclusion

PEH treatment is challenging, as this disease tends to occur in more complex elderly patients who often present with multiple medical problems and a variety of associated symptoms. The preoperative evaluation is an important component in the preparation of a safe and effective operative strategy. There are many advantages of utilizing the laparoscopic approach to PEH repair, including decreased hospital length of stay, improved recovery time, and decreased complications. Some studies have shown that laparoscopic PEH repair may have a higher incidence of hernia recurrence, but the full clinical significance of these recurrences is unknown. In order to maximize the efficacy of this procedure, modifications such as performing a fundoplication and using an absorbable mesh onlay to reinforce the cruroplasty have emerged. Though more prospective, randomized studies are needed to support the superior results of these surgical adjuncts, laparoscopic PEH repair with an anti-reflux procedure and absorbable mesh should be the current standard of care.

References

1. Stylopoulos N, Rattner DW. The history of hiatal hernia surgery: from Bowditch to laparoscopy. Ann Surg. 2005;241(1):185–93.
2. Mittal RK. Hiatal hernia. Am J Med. 1997;103(5):33S–9S.
3. Oleynikov D, Ranade A, Parcells J, Bills N. Paraesophageal hernias and Nissen fundoplication. In: Oleynikov D, Bills N, editors. Robotic surgery for the general surgeon. 1st ed. Hauppauge: Nova Biomedical; 2014. p. 65–74.
4. Tiwari MM, Tsang AW, Reynoso JF, Oleynikov D. Options for large hiatal defects. In: Murayama K, Chand B, Kothari S, Mikami D, Nagle A, editors. Evidence-based approach to minimally invasive surgery. 1st ed. Woodbury: Cine-Med, Incorporated; 2011.
5. El Sherif A, Yano F, Mittal S, Filipi CJ. Collagen metabolism and recurrent hiatal hernia: cause and effect? Hernia. 2006;10(6):511–20.
6. Arafat FO, Teitelbaum EN, Hungness ES. Modern treatment of paraesophageal hernia: preoperative evaluation and technique for laparoscopic repair. Surg Laparosc Endosc Percutan Tech. 2012;22(4):297–303.
7. Maganty K, Smith RL. Cameron lesions: unusual cause of gastrointestinal bleeding and anemia. Digestion. 2008;77(3–4):214–7.
8. Auyang ED, Oelschlager BK. Laparoscopic paraesophageal hernia repair. In: Swanstrom L, Soper N, editors. Mastery of endoscopic and laparoscopic surgery. 4th ed. Philadelphia: Lippincott Williams & Wilkins; 2013. p. 65–74.
9. O'Rourke RW, Khajanchee YS, Urbach DR, Lee NN, Lockhart B, Hansen PD, et al. Extended transmediastinal dissection: an alternative to gastroplasty for short esophagus. Arch Surg. 2003;138(7):735–40.
10. Bochkarev V, Lee YK, Vitamvas M, Oleynikov D. Short esophagus: how much length can we get? Surg Endosc. 2008;22(10):2123–7.
11. Draaisma W, Gooszen H, Tournoij E, Broeders I. Controversies in paraesophageal hernia repair; a review of literature. Surg Endosc. 2005;19(10):1300–8.
12. Lebenthal A, Waterford SD, Fisichella PM. Treatment and controversies in paraesophageal hernia repair. Front Surg. 2015;2:13.
13. Daigle CR, Funch-Jensen P, Calatayud D, Rask P, Jacobsen B, Grantcharov TP. Laparoscopic repair of paraesophageal hernia with anterior gastropexy: a multicenter study. Surg Endosc. 2015;29(7):1856–61.
14. DeMeester SR. Laparoscopic paraesophageal hernia repair: critical steps and adjunct techniques to minimize recurrence. Surg Laparosc Endosc Percutan Tech. 2013;23(5):429–35.
15. Soper NJ, Teitelbaum EN. Laparoscopic paraesophageal hernia repair: current controversies. Surg Laparosc Endosc Percutan Tech. 2013;23(5):442–5.
16. Stefanidis D, Hope WW, Kohn GP, Reardon PR, Richardson WS, Fanelli RD, et al. Guidelines for surgical treatment of gastroesophageal reflux disease. Surg Endosc. 2010;24(11):2647–69.
17. Granderath F, Carlson M, Champion J, Szold A, Basso N, Pointner R, et al. Prosthetic closure of the esophageal hiatus in large hiatal hernia repair and laparoscopic antireflux surgery. Surg Endosc. 2006;20(3):367–79.
18. Davis SS. Current controversies in paraesophageal hernia repair. Surg Clin North Am. 2008;88(5):959–78.
19. Antoniou SA, Pointner R, Granderath FA. Hiatal hernia repair with the use of biologic meshes: a literature review. Surg Laparosc Endosc Percutan Tech. 2011;21(1):1–9.
20. Stadlhuber RJ, El Sherif A, Mittal SK, Fitzgibbons RJ, Brunt LM, Hunter JG, et al. Mesh complications after prosthetic reinforcement of hiatal closure: a 28-case series. Surg Endosc. 2009;23(6):1219–26.
21. Oelschlager BK, Barreca M, Chang L, Pellegrini CA. The use of small intestine submucosa in the repair of paraesophageal hernias: initial observations of a new technique. Am J Surg. 2003;186(1):4–8.

22. Schmidt E, Shaligram A, Reynoso JF, Kothari V, Oleynikov D. Hiatal hernia repair with bio-logic mesh reinforcement reduces recurrence rate in small hiatal hernias. Dis Esophagus. 2014;27(1):13–7.
23. Lee YK, James E, Bochkarev V, Vitamvas M, Oleynikov D. Long-term outcome of cruroplasty reinforcement with human acellular dermal matrix in large paraesophageal hiatal hernia. J Gastrointest Surg. 2008;12(5):811–5.
24. Poncet G, Robert M, Roman S, Boulez J. Laparoscopic repair of large hiatal hernia without prosthetic reinforcement: late results and relevance of anterior gastropexy. J Gastrointest Surg. 2010;14(12):1910–6.
25. Higashi S, Nakajima K, Tanaka K, Miyazaki Y, Makino T, Takahashi T, et al. Laparoscopic ante-rior gastropexy for type III/IV hiatal hernia in elderly patients. Surg Case Rep. 2017;3(1):45.

Short Esophagus

8

Takahiro Masuda and Sumeet K. Mittal

Introduction

For an antireflux surgery to be successful, it should include fundoplication around the distal esophagus, which lies tension-free below the diaphragm. In order to carry out a tension-free repair, however, 2–3 cm of intra-diaphragmatic esophageal length is required. A short esophagus (SE) is a well-recognized risk factor for failure of an antireflux procedure, and although this concept may seem straightforward, it is nonetheless controversial. Most surgeons believe that a subset of patients will be found to have SE intraoperatively, but no uniformly accepted definition of SE yet exists—resulting in great variation in preoperative and intraoperative protocols for SE. Some argue that the esophagus can simply be mobilized to achieve adequate length for a tension-free repair [1–3]; others propose anchoring the gastroesophageal junction (GEJ) to the arcuate ligament to obtain sufficient esophageal length for a fundoplication.

The essential concept of SE is that adequate intra-abdominal esophageal length cannot be achieved even after maximal esophageal mobilization. By definition, then, an SE can only be diagnosed intraoperatively—after complete esophageal mobilization [4]. Again, this is subject to some ambiguity (e.g., How much caudad traction should there be at the GEJ when assessing the length of the intra-abdominal esophagus?) [5]. Any preoperative findings, including the size of a hiatal hernia, presence of Barrett's esophagus or esophageal stricture, and manometric esophageal length, are risk factors for SE; however, they are not signs that allow for definitive SE diagnosis. Most centers report the prevalence of SE between 3% and 14% in patients undergoing primary antireflux surgery [4–9]. Well-known risk factors for

T. Masuda, M.D. · S. K. Mittal, M.D. (✉)
Norton Thoracic Institute, St. Joseph's Hospital and Medical Center, Phoenix, AZ, USA

Creighton University School of Medicine, Phoenix Regional Campus, Phoenix, AZ, USA
e-mail: Sumeet.Mittal@DignityHealth.org

© Springer International Publishing AG, part of Springer Nature 2018
D. Oleynikov, P. M. Fisichella (eds.), *A Mastery Approach to Complex Esophageal Diseases*, https://doi.org/10.1007/978-3-319-75795-7_8

SE include: more than 5 cm between the GEJ and hiatus on contrast esophagram, a short manometric intrasphincteric esophageal length, a long segment of Barrett's esophagus, and distal esophageal stricture. Failure to recognize an SE may result in tension at the fundoplication or creation of a fundoplication around the proximal stomach. If an SE goes unrecognized and a fundoplication is carried out without a lengthening procedure, the risk of surgical failure (e.g., a slipped fundoplication and crural disruption), is increased due to excessive tension on the wrap [4, 10]. Redo antireflux surgery carries higher rates of intraoperative complications and poorer outcomes than primary surgery [11]. Unrecognized SE is believed to account for 20% to 43% of all surgical failures after open or laparoscopic antireflux surgery [4, 12]. Therefore, SE management in primary surgery is of great clinical importance.

Pathophysiology

Short esophagus is a complication of long-term inflammation in the esophageal wall induced by chronic gastroesophageal reflux disease (GERD) [4, 13]. Repeated chemical esophageal injury due to acid or alkaline refluxate can lead to panmural inflammatory cell infiltration. Then, recurrent episodes of reflux-induced inflammatory responses result in irreversible fibrosis and scarring secondary to the healing process. This transmural esophageal fibrosis of the longitudinal muscles produces esophageal shortening; meanwhile, circumferential scarring of the esophageal mucosa, submucosa, and circular fibers leads to peptic stricture [14].

The severity of peptic stricture and the degree of esophageal shortening go hand-in-hand. Several studies have reported peptic stricture as a risk factor for SE [15, 16]. Interestingly, recently published reports have shown that the severity and incidence of esophagitis are statistically similar in preoperative endoscopic evaluations between patients with and without SE who underwent antireflux surgery [15, 17]. The incidence of SE has been declining, which may be a result of widespread use of the acid suppression therapy that decreases the degree of acid-induced esophageal damage.

Assessment

Preoperative Assessment

The ability to predict an SE preoperatively helps surgeons avoid unplanned, complex procedures. Various studies of preoperative evaluations have been aimed at identifying an SE, including barium esophagram, esophagogastroduodenoscopy, and esophageal manometry [7, 8, 15–19]. Our group has previously assessed the predictability of intraoperative SE diagnosis based upon commonly accepted criteria of preoperative SE indicators, including: (1) hiatal hernia ≥5 cm or large paraesophageal hernia on upright esophagram, (2) stricture formation or Barrett's esophagus on endoscopic evaluation, and (3) short esophageal length on manometric analysis (defined as two standard deviations below the mean for height) [8]. Each parameter had low positive predictive value (PPV)—less than 40%.

Investigating a larger sample size ($n = 260$), Awad et al. [19] reported the predictive utility of those three preoperative studies (i.e., esophagram, endoscopy, and manometry) both individually and in conjunction with one another. They confirmed that individual risk factors had low PPV (again, less than 40%). Endoscopic evaluation alone had the highest sensitivity rate for SE (61%), but it also had the lowest specificity (42%). The combination of two or more tests increased specificity (63–100%), which resulted in low sensitivity (28–42%). Awad et al. [19] therefore concluded that the best screening test for SE may be endoscopy, but no ideal predictive test is apparent.

Recently, Yano et al. [15] suggested that preoperative endoscopic finding only has a high reliability in identifying patients' risk of SE, but not diagnosing actual SE. They defined an esophageal length index (ELI): the ratio of endoscopic esophageal length (cm) to patient height (meters), and showed that the cutoff value of ELI ≤19.5 had a specificity of 95%, a PPV of 81%, and a negative predictive value of 83%, although sensitivity was as low as 56%. The ELI seems to be the most useful current tool for identifying patients who will not need a lengthening procedure (false negative rate: 19%). However, the low true-positive rate makes it difficult to determine which patients will be more likely to require an intraoperative lengthening procedure. No absolute diagnostic test can predict SE preoperatively.

Intraoperative Assessment

The gold standard for diagnosis of SE is intraoperative assessment of the intra-abdominal esophageal length after complete mobilization of the esophagus [8]. The intra-abdominal length of the esophagus is measured as the distance from arch of the crus to the GEJ. The GEJ is identified by skeletonization of the angle of His, and can be localized with intraoperative endoscopy. The generally agreed-upon length of intra-abdominal esophagus for a tension-free fundoplication is 2–3 cm [4, 7, 8, 13, 18, 20].

Surgical approach and degree of esophageal mobilization have tremendous effects on the measurement of the intra-abdominal esophagus [5]. In the era of laparoscopic surgery, esophageal mobilization via the transhiatal approach is feasible and safe. Various surgeons have described a sufficient degree of esophageal mobilization under transhiatal laparoscopic control. Horvath et al. [4] suggested that if the distal 3–4 cm of esophagus is circumferentially mobilized and sufficient intra-abdominal esophageal length still cannot be obtained, the esophageal dissection should be extended to the mediastinum. Johnson et al. [7] described carrying out the dissection into the mediastinum for 4–6 cm, and O'Rourke et al. [21] extended the dissection anywhere between 7 and 10 cm into the mediastinum. Furthermore, Bochkarev et al. [22] reported safe mediastinal dissection up to 18 cm under laparoscopic control—but because that implies dissection nearly to the thoracic inlet, this claim should be taken with a grain of salt.

The above review implies that, with the refinement of laparoscopic esophageal surgery, surgeons can extend the maximal length of esophageal mobilization. However, it is best to proceed conservatively, mobilizing circumferentially and assessing intra-abdominal esophageal length until adequate esophageal length is achieved or until the surgeon has reached his or her technical limit. In our practice, we perform mediastinal dissection to mobilize the esophagus circumferentially to a height of at least 8 cm above the hiatus [23].

DeMeester et al. [24] carried out a swine study in which they compared laparoscopic and transthoracic procedures to determine which approach resulted in a greater increase in esophageal length. They found that transthoracic mobilization produced a longer intra-abdominal esophageal length, even after maximal mobilization with laparoscopic surgery. DeMeester et al. [24] therefore recommend that, in situations in which laparoscopic mobilization alone does not garner adequate intra-abdominal length, transthoracic mobilization should be considered.

Surgical Treatment Options

Primary Surgery for Short Esophagus

Various surgical options for SE have been reported, including intrathoracic fundoplication, esophageal resection, and lengthening procedures. Intrathoracic fundoplication has been reported to provide relief from reflux [25]; however, it is associated with unacceptably high rate of severe postoperative complications, such as ulceration, hemorrhage, strangulation, and intrathoracic rupture of the gastric wrap [26, 27]. Another option is esophageal resection and reconstruction of the upper digestive tract using the stomach, jejunum, or colon [25]. Esophageal resection with reconstruction is undoubtedly a challenging, extensive procedure; however, it has been associated with good symptomatic and functional outcomes in patients with advanced GERD who present with dysphagia in the setting of SE and poor esophageal motility [6]. The most common treatment for SE is an esophageal lengthening procedure in the form of a cut Collis gastroplasty with fundoplication.

In 1957, Collis [28] described a gastroplasty for hiatal hernia with SE to avoid esophagectomy. The operation was performed through an abdominothoracic incision. After dissection of the mediastinum, an esophageal dilator was placed per orally into the stomach. The proximal stomach was divided parallel to the dilator, creating a neoesophagus (Fig. 8.1). Although Collis himself did not add a fundoplication, the neoesophagus allowed a tension-free fundoplication, as represented by the Collis-Belsey procedure [29].

The advent of minimally invasive surgery has revolutionized antireflux surgery, including the Collis gastroplasty. Swanstrom et al. [18] first reported carrying out a laparoscopic Collis-Nissen procedure with right thoracoscopy in 1996. In their approach, a 3-cm endoscopic linear stapling device was introduced through a 12-mm trocar placed in the right chest, passed transhiatally into the abdomen, and positioned parallel to and above the esophagus (Fig. 8.2a). The proximal stomach

Fig. 8.1 Collis
gastroplasty. *Used with
permission from Norton
Thoracic Institute,
Phoenix, Arizona*

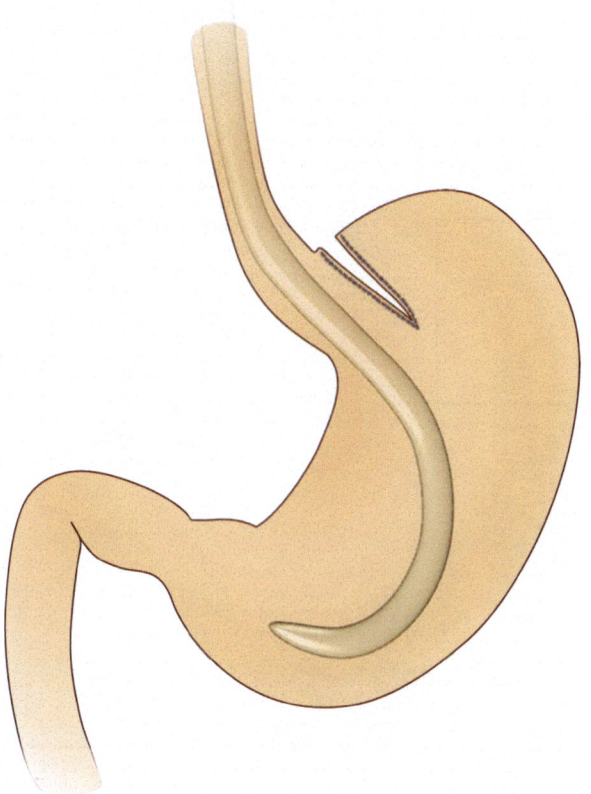

was "fed" in to the stapler with a bougie *in situ*. Firing the stapler created a cut
Collis gastroplasty, and a fundoplication was created around the neoesophagus.

Johnson et al. [7] described the first totally laparoscopic technique for SE in 1998.
They adapted an open approach (previously described by Steichen [30]) into a laparoscopic procedure. In this method, creation of a neoesophagus required two different
stapling devices. These surgeons used a 21-mm circular stapling device to create a
sealed window through both the anterior and posterior gastric walls at the assumed
lower end of the neoesophagus. A 3-cm endoscopic linear stapler was then placed
through this transgastric window and fired toward the angle of His (Fig. 8.2b). The
resulting neoesophagus facilitated a tension-free fundoplication. Terry et al. [31] later
reported that this dual-stapler procedure introduced the possibility of tissue ischemia at
the apex of the fundus, and suggested that a stapled-wedge Collis gastroplasty may be
superior in terms of avoiding tissue ischemia and reducing operative time and morbidity (Fig. 8.2c).

The development of the articulating endoscopic linear stapler has allowed surgeons to perform safer, more effective procedures in the setting of SE. In 2000, our
group first reported a left-sided, thoracoscopically assisted laparoscopic Collis gastroplasty [20]. The technique for this surgical procedure is described in detail below.

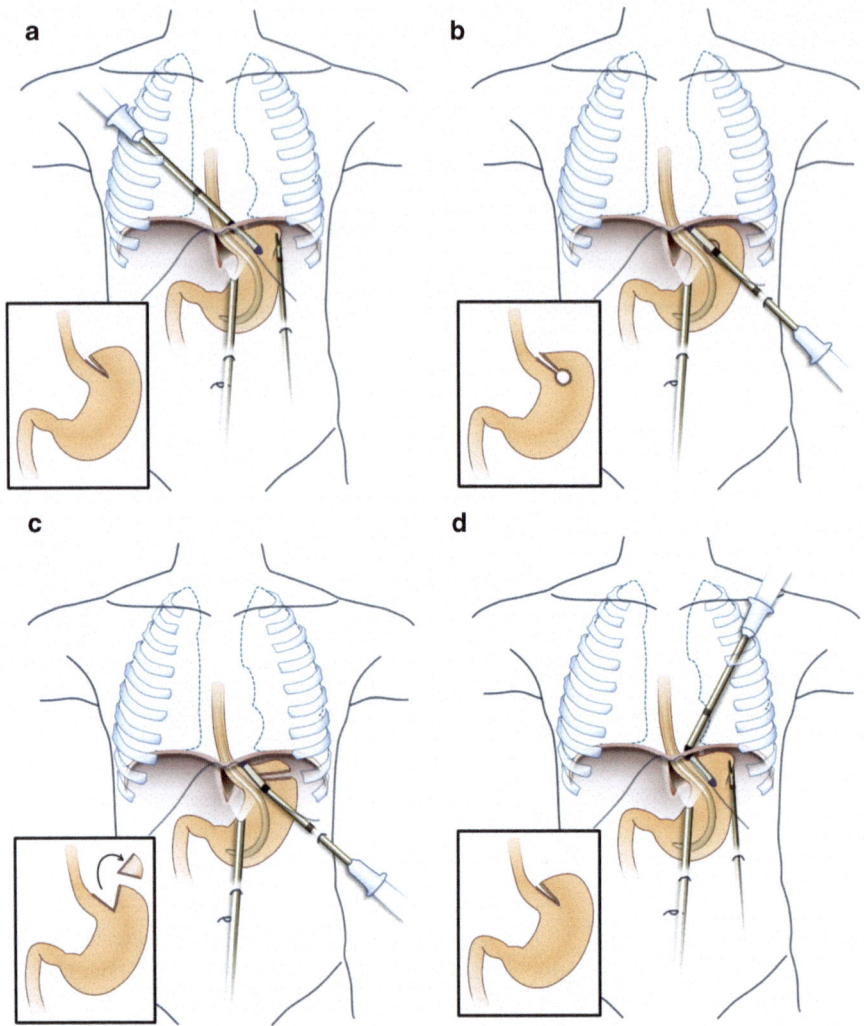

Fig. 8.2 (**a**) Right-sided, thoracoscopically assisted laparoscopic Collis gastroplasty. (**b**) Double-stapled laparoscopic Collis gastroplasty. (**c**) Stapled-wedge laparoscopic Collis gastroplasty. (**d**) Left-sided, thoracoscopically assisted laparoscopic Collis gastroplasty. *Used with permission from Norton Thoracic Institute, Phoenix, Arizona*

Left-Sided, Thoracoscopically Assisted Laparoscopic Collis-Nissen Procedure

The patient is placed in the lithotomy position. After general anesthesia, the left arm is placed on an arm board. The abdomen and left chest are prepped for surgery. Five ports are placed in the standard locations, as for laparoscopic Nissen fundoplication

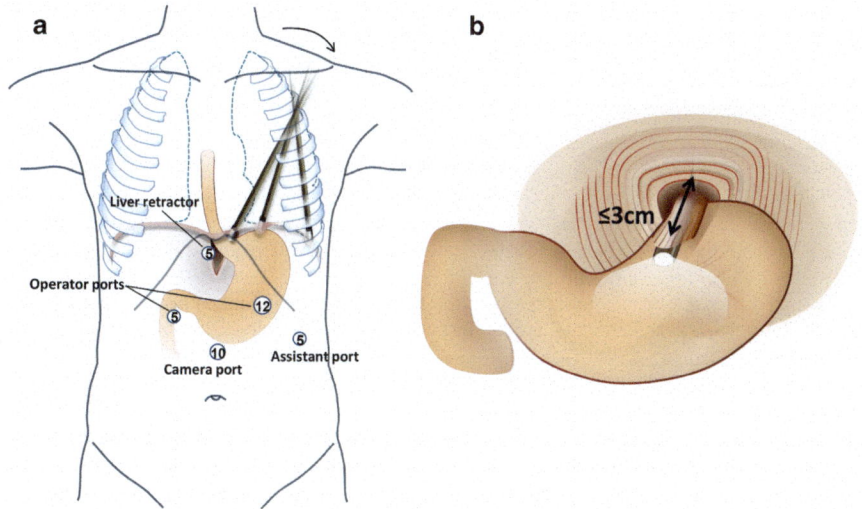

Fig. 8.3 (a) Five ports are placed in the standard locations. A blunt probe is advanced into the left thoracic cavity, and walked toward the hiatus. (b) An intra-abdominal esophageal length of less than 3 cm is deemed a "short esophagus." Used with permission from Norton Thoracic Institute, Phoenix, Arizona

(Fig. 8.3a). The short gastric vessels are divided routinely. After the hiatus is freed, mediastinal dissection is performed to mobilize the esophagus circumferentially to a height of at least 8 cm above the hiatus. Skeletonization of the angle of His is performed, and great care must be taken to avoid injuring the vagus nerve. The intra-abdominal length of the esophagus is then assessed as the distance between the arch of the crus and the GEJ (intraoperative endoscopy often proves extremely useful in identifying the GEJ). A patient is determined to have an SE if this distance measures less than 3 cm (Fig. 8.3b).

A 3–4 cm incision is made at the left anterior axillary line, between the 3rd and 4th intercostal spaces, according to individual variability of anatomical chest shape (higher is better). Before the linear stapler is inserted, a blunt probe is advanced into the left thoracic cavity (Fig. 8.3a). This probe is pushed against the left hemidiaphragm and is visualized laparoscopically as a diaphragmatic indentation. The probe tip is "walked" toward the hiatus and bluntly penetrates the mediastinal pleura, entering the abdominal cavity. After accessibility to the abdominal cavity is deemed safe, the probe is removed. This technique does not require thoracoscopic visual guidance.

Using the same technique, an articulating linear stapler (EndoGIA, Ethicon, New Brunswick, NJ) 30–45 mm in length is inserted and "walked" across the diaphragm. It is placed through the hiatus, into the peritoneal cavity. The stapler is articulated to lay parallel to the esophagus and is placed just to the left of the angle of His. The greater curvature of the stomach is advanced into the open jaws of the stapler.

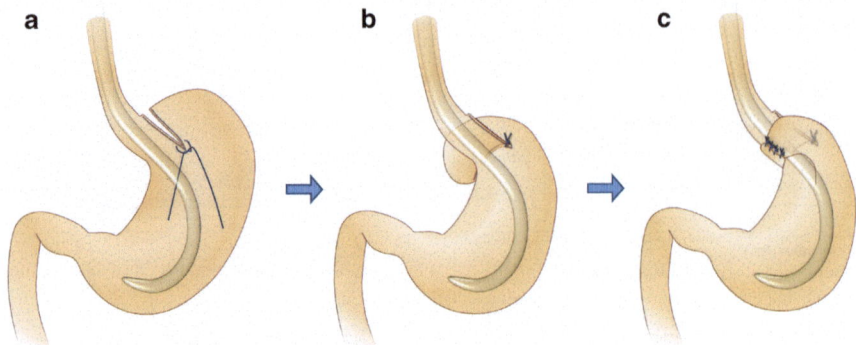

Fig. 8.4 Floppy Nissen fundoplication around the neoesophagus. *Used with permission from Norton Thoracic Institute, Phoenix, Arizona*

A 46-Fr bougie is passed down the esophagus and into the stomach to ensure the diameter of the neoesophagus is adequate (Fig. 8.2d). The stapler is fired and removed. If additional stapling is required to obtain adequate length of the Collis segment, the above steps are repeated. A chest tube is then placed, and crural closure is performed. A single 3–0 silk suture is placed at the bifurcation point of the two staple lines (Fig. 8.4a) to prevent excess tension at the staple line. The fundus is wrapped around the neoesophagus (Fig. 8.4b, c), and a standard Nissen, floppy Nissen, or Toupet fundoplication is performed.

Reoperation for Previously Unrecognized Short Esophagus

A subset of patients who require a reoperative antireflux procedure have an SE that went undetected at the time of the primary surgery. Our group has reported that 13–15% of patients who undergo reoperative antireflux surgery were found to have an SE, and therefore required Collis gastroplasty [23, 32]. In such patients, the esophageal length was assessed after the fundoplication was dismantled and the mediastinum was mobilized.

Collis gastroplasty with redo fundoplication is the most common reoperative intervention for a previously unrecognized SE. If an SE is assessed after fundoplication takedown and esophageal mobilization, a Collis gastroplasty followed by fundoplication is performed (described above). However, some patients experience poor outcomes with redo Collis gastroplasty, particularly if they have esophageal stricture that cannot be dilated, very poor esophageal motility secondary to chronic GERD, or both. In such patients, redo fundoplication may cause severe dysphagia. Patients who have a scarred fundus, morbid obesity, or delayed gastric emptying may also be at risk of poor surgical outcomes after Collis–fundoplication. For patients who require antireflux surgery but also have these risk factors, we recommend Roux-en-Y (RNY) reconstruction with esophagojejunostomy (EJ) or gastrojejunostomy (GJ) [33–35].

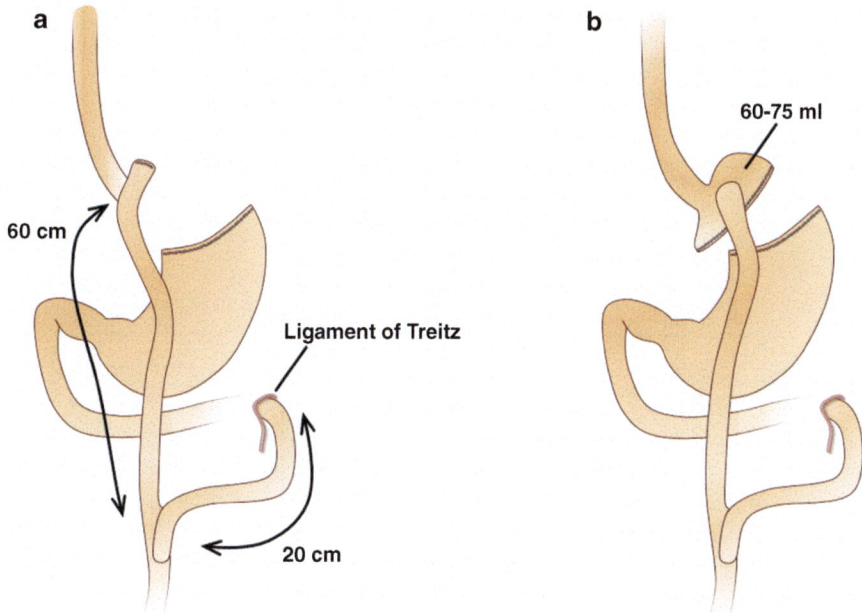

Fig. 8.5 Roux-en-Y (RNY) reconstruction. (**a**) RNY esophagojejunostomy. (**b**) RNY gastrojeju-nostomy. *Used with permission from Norton Thoracic Institute, Phoenix, Arizona*

In patients with an SE, either a RNY–EJ (for esophageal stricture that cannot be dilated) or RNY–GJ (for esophageal dysmotility) is recommended. RNY reconstruction allows near-complete diversion of both the gastric and duodenal refluxate from the esophagus without risking outflow obstruction secondary to a too-tight fundoplication.

Roux-en-Y Reconstruction Technique

After dismantling the previous fundoplication and crural repair, the esophagus (above the stricture, if stricture is present) or stomach (to create a 60–100-cc pouch based on lesser curvature) is created using linear staplers. The distal stomach is left *in situ*. The alimentary and biliary limbs are tailored to 60 cm and 20 cm in length, respectively, and RNY anastomosis is completed (Fig. 8.5a, b). A gastrostomy tube is placed, especially if the patient is malnourished, is taking medications that need to be continued in the perioperative period, or both.

Outcomes of Surgical Treatments

Before the advent of minimally invasive surgery, open Collis gastroplasty with fundo-plication was associated with excellent results in 75–93% of patients over the long-term follow-up period [36–38]. Several investigators later described similar

Table 8.1 Outcomes of Collis gastroplasty with fundoplication

Author, year	n	Approach	Follow-up period	Good or excellent results (%)	Morbidity (%)	Leak (%)	Recurrent objective reflux (%)	Postoperative reflux symptoms (%)	Postoperative dysphagia (%)	Recurrent hiatal hernia (%)	Required reoperation (%)	Mortality (%)
Henderson (1985) [38]	335	Open	5–8.5 years	93.1	N/A	0.9	0	2.9	0	1.1	N/A	0
Stirling (1989) [37]	261	Open	1–11 years	75	7.9	1.7	9	25	42	N/A	10	1.1
Richardson (1998) [36]	52	Open	1–18 years	92.3	26.9	0	N/A	5.8	75	13.5	0	0
Jobe (1998) [13]	14	Lap	14 months	N/A	21.4	0	50	14	14	0	0	0
Awad (2000) [20]	8	Lap	9–34 months	87.5	50	0	N/A	12.5	N/A	N/A	N/A	0
Houghton (2008) [39]	116	Open/Lap	1–70 months	84	18	3	N/A	10.1	19.1	3	3	0
Garg (2009) [23]	85	Open/Lap	9–111 months	76.9	30.6	2.4	N/A	24	28	N/A	4.7	0
Nason (2011) [40]	454	Lap	33 months (median) 3333 months (median)	93	20	2.7	N/A	24.8	27.6	16.6	2.7	1.5
Zehetner (2014) [41]	85	Lap	12 months (median)	N/A	8	0	11	7	16	2.4	N/A	0

Lap Laparoscopy, *N/A* Not applicable

postoperative satisfaction between laparoscopic and open surgical cohorts [23, 39]. Nowadays, the laparoscopic approach is the preferred method. The existing literature on outcomes of Collis gastroplasty with fundoplication is summarized in Table 8.1.

Perioperative morbidity is reported to be approximately 10–30% and includes atelectasis, atrial fibrillation, ileus, pneumonia, urinary tract infection, pneumothorax, pleural effusion, and postoperative leak [13, 20, 23, 36–41]. A staple-line leak has been reported in 2–3% of patients who undergo laparoscopic Collis–fundoplication, but less than 2% of patients who underwent an open approach developed staple-line leaks [13, 20, 23, 36–41]. Nason et al. [40] described more postoperative leaks in the dual-stapler procedure (Fig. 8.2b) than in the wedge-Collis procedure (Fig. 8.2c), but this difference was not statistically significant (3.1% vs. 1.6%). Recurring hiatal hernia occurs in 0–17% of patients (including small hiatal hernia; Table 8.1). Postoperative reflux symptoms are seen in 3–25% of patients—a rate similar to that found in patients who undergo standard fundoplication without an SE. The incidence of postoperative dysphagia is very wide, occurring in 0–75% of patients, depending on the preoperative presence of esophageal stricture. Mortality is very low across the board.

Although symptoms and quality of life are dramatically improved after surgery, some studies have shown disparity between subjective and objective outcomes [13, 42, 43]. Jobe et al. [13] found that 50% of patients who underwent laparoscopic Collis gastroplasty with fundoplication had abnormal results on 24-hour pH study (the average DeMeester score in these patients was 100), despite the fact that 71.4% (5/7) of these patients did not experience postoperative heartburn. They suggested that the postoperative abnormal acid exposure may have been caused by neoesophageal acid secreting on the oral side of the fundoplication, coupled with poor acid clearance due to the aperistaltic neoesophagus. Mor et al. [44] found that the acid clearance time was significantly longer in patients who underwent a Collis–Nissen procedure than it was in healthy controls or in patients who underwent Nissen fundoplication alone.

Some surgeons have suggested that if a tension-free fundoplication could be created that also avoids acid-secreting mucosa proximal to the wrap, good physiologic outcomes with favorable symptomatic results may result [31, 42, 44]. However, it is impossible to keep the fundoplication on the oral side of the neoesophagus in some patients with an SE, because the Collis gastroplasty can extend above the hiatus in these patients. In such complex cases, RNY reconstruction may be a more attractive alternative.

References

1. Coster DD, Bower WH, Wilson VT, Brebrick RT, Richardson GL. Laparoscopic partial fundoplication vs laparoscopic Nissen-Rosetti fundoplication. Short-term results of 231 cases. Surg Endosc. 1997;11:625–31.
2. Madan AK, Frantzides CT, Patsavas KL. The myth of the short esophagus. Surg Endosc. 2004;18:31–4.

3. Korn O, Csendes A, Burdiles P, Braghetto I, Sagastume H, Biagini L. Length of the esophagus in patients with gastroesophageal reflux disease and Barrett's esophagus compared to controls. Surgery. 2003;133:358–63.
4. Horvath KD, Swanstrom LL, Jobe BA. The short esophagus: pathophysiology, incidence, presentation, and treatment in the era of laparoscopic antireflux surgery. Ann Surg. 2000;232:630–40.
5. DeMeester SR, DeMeester TR. Editorial comment: The short esophagus: going, going, gone? Surgery. 2003;133:364–7.
6. Ritter MP, Peters JH, DeMeester TR, Gadenstätter M, Oberg S, Fein M, Hagen JA, Crookes PF, Bremner CG. Treatment of advanced gastroesophageal reflux disease with Collis gastroplasty and Belsey partial fundoplication. Arch Surg. 1998;133:523–8. discussion 528–529
7. Johnson AB, Oddsdottir M, Hunter JG. Laparoscopic Collis gastroplasty and Nissen fundoplication. A new technique for the management of esophageal foreshortening. Surg Endosc. 1998;12:1055–60.
8. Mittal SK, Awad ZT, Tasset M, Filipi CJ, Dickason TJ, Shinno Y, Marsh RE, Tomonaga TJ, Lerner C. The preoperative predictability of the short esophagus in patients with stricture or paraesophageal hernia. Surg Endosc. 2000;14:464–8.
9. Awad ZT, Filipi CJ. The short esophagus: pathogenesis, diagnosis, and current surgical options. Arch Surg. 2001;136:113–4.
10. Awad ZT, Anderson PI, Sato K, Roth TA, Gerhardt J, Filipi CJ. Laparoscopic reoperative antireflux surgery. Surg Endosc. 2001;15:1401–7.
11. Grover BT, Kothari SN. Reoperative antireflux surgery. Surg Clin North Am. 2015;95:629–40.
12. Awais O, Luketich JD, Schuchert MJ, Morse CR, Wilson J, Gooding WE, Landreneau RJ, Pennathur A. Reoperative antireflux surgery for failed fundoplication: an analysis of outcomes in 275 patients. Ann Thorac Surg. 2011;92:1083–9. discussion 1089–1090.
13. Jobe BA, Horvath KD, Swanstrom LL. Postoperative function following laparoscopic collis gastroplasty for shortened esophagus. Arch Surg. 1998;133:867–74.
14. Kunio NR, Dolan JP, Hunter JG. Short esophagus. Surg Clin North Am. 2015;95:641–52.
15. Yano F, Stadlhuber RJ, Tsuboi K, Garg N, Filipi CJ, Mittal SK. Preoperative predictability of the short esophagus: endoscopic criteria. Surg Endosc. 2009;23:1308–12.
16. Gastal OL, Hagen JA, Peters JH, Campos GM, Hashemi M, Theisen J, Bremner CG, DeMeester TR. Short esophagus: analysis of predictors and clinical implications. Arch Surg. 1999;134:633–6. discussion 637–638.
17. Durand L, De Antón R, Caracoche M, Covián E, Gimenez M, Ferraina P, Swanström L. Short esophagus: selection of patients for surgery and long-term results. Surg Endosc. 2012;26:704–13.
18. Swanstrom LL, Marcus DR, Galloway GQ. Laparoscopic Collis gastroplasty is the treatment of choice for the shortened esophagus. Am J Surg. 1996;171:477–81.
19. Awad ZT, Mittal SK, Roth TA, Anderson PI, Wilfley WA Jr, Filipi CJ. Esophageal shortening during the era of laparoscopic surgery. World J Surg. 2001;25:558–61.
20. Awad ZT, Filipi CJ, Mittal SK, Roth TA, Marsh RE, Shiino Y, Tomonaga T. Left side thoracoscopically assisted gastroplasty: a new technique for managing the shortened esophagus. Surg Endosc. 2000;14:508–12.
21. O'Rourke RW, Khajanchee YS, Urbach DR, Lee NN, Lockhart B, Hansen PD, Swanstrom LL. Extended transmediastinal dissection: an alternative to gastroplasty for short esophagus. Arch Surg. 2003;138:735–40.
22. Bochkarev V, Lee YK, Vitamvas M, Oleynikov D. Short esophagus: how much length can we get? Surg Endosc. 2008;22:2123–7.
23. Garg N, Yano F, Filipi CJ, Mittal SK. Long-term symptomatic outcomes after Collis gastroplasty with fundoplication. Dis Esophagus. 2009;22:532–8.
24. DeMeester SR, Sillin LF, Lin HW, Gurski RR. Increasing esophageal length: a comparison of laparoscopic versus transthoracic esophageal mobilization with and without vagal trunk division in pigs. J Am Coll Surg. 2003;197:558–64.

25. Moghissi K. Intrathoracic fundoplication for reflux stricture associated with short oesophagus. Thorax. 1983;38:36–40.
26. Richardson JD, Larson GM, Polk HC Jr. Intrathoracic fundoplication for shortened esophagus. Treacherous solution to a challenging problem. Am J Surg. 1982;143:29–35.
27. Mansour KA, Burton HG, Miller JI Jr, Hatcher CR Jr. Complications of intrathoracic Nissen fundoplication. Ann Thorac Surg. 1981;32:173–8.
28. Collis JL. An operation for hiatus hernia with short oesophagus. Thorax. 1957;12:181–8.
29. Pearson FG, Langer B, Henderson RD. Gastroplasty and Belsey hiatus hernia repair. An operation for the management of peptic stricture with acquired short esophagus. J Thorac Cardiovasc Surg. 1971;61:50–63.
30. Steichen FM. Abdominal approach to the Collis gastroplasty and Nissen fundoplication. Surg Gynecol Obstet. 1986;162:272–4.
31. Terry ML, Vernon A, Hunter JG. Stapled-wedge Collis gastroplasty for the shortened esophagus. Am J Surg. 2004;188:195–9.
32. Iqbal A, Awad Z, Simkins J, Shah R, Haider M, Salinas V, Turaga K, Karu A, Mittal SK, Filipi CJ. Repair of 104 failed anti-reflux operations. Ann Surg. 2006;244:42–51.
33. Makris KI, Lee T, Mittal SK. Roux-en-Y reconstruction for failed fundoplication. J Gastrointest Surg. 2009;13:2226–32.
34. Makris KI, Panwar A, Willer BL, Ali A, Sramek KL, Lee TH, Mittal SK. The role of short-limb Roux-en-Y reconstruction for failed antireflux surgery: a single-center 5-year experience. Surg Endosc. 2012;26:1279–86.
35. Mittal SK, Légner A, Tsuboi K, Juhasz A, Bathla L, Lee TH. Roux-en-Y reconstruction is superior to redo fundoplication in a subset of patients with failed antireflux surgery. Surg Endosc. 2013;27:927–35.
36. Richardson JD, Richardson RL. Collis-Nissen gastroplasty for shortened esophagus: long-term evaluation. Ann Surg. 1998;227:735–40. discussion 740–742.
37. Stirling MC, Orringer MB. Continued assessment of the combined Collis-Nissen operation. Ann Thorac Surg. 1989;47:224–30.
38. Henderson RD, Marryatt GV. Total fundoplication gastroplasty (Nissen gastroplasty): five-year review. Ann Thorac Surg. 1985;39:74–9.
39. Houghton SG, Deschamps C, Cassivi SD, Allen MS, Nichols FC 3rd, Barnes SA, Pairolero PC. Combined transabdominal gastroplasty and fundoplication for shortened esophagus: impact on reflux-related and overall quality of life. Ann Thorac Surg. 2008;85:1947–52.
40. Nason KS, Luketich JD, Awais O, Abbas G, Pennathur A, Landreneau RJ, Schuchert MJ. Quality of life after collis gastroplasty for short esophagus in patients with paraesophageal hernia. Ann Thorac Surg. 2011;92:1854–60. discussion 1860–1861.
41. Zehetner J, DeMeester SR, Ayazi S, Kilday P, Alicuben ET, DeMeester TR. Laparoscopic wedge fundectomy for collis gastroplasty creation in patients with a foreshortened esophagus. Ann Surg. 2014;260:1030–3.
42. Tsuboi K, Omura N, Kashiwagi H, Yano F, Ishibashi Y, Suzuki Y, Kawasaki N, Mitsumori N, Urashima M, Yanaga K. Laparoscopic Collis gastroplasty and Nissen fundoplication for reflux esophagitis with shortened esophagus in Japanese patients. Surg Laparosc Endosc Percutan Tech. 2006;16:401–5.
43. Martin CJ, Cox MR, Cade RJ. Collis-Nissen gastroplasty fundoplication for complicated gastro-oesophageal reflux disease. Aust N Z J Surg. 1992;62:126–9.
44. Mor A, Lutfi R, Torquati A. Esophageal acid-clearance physiology is altered after Nissen-Collis gastroplasty. Surg Endosc. 2013;27:1334–8.

Benign Esophageal Tumors

9

Emanuele Asti, Stefano Siboni, and Luigi Bonavina

Introduction

Benign esophageal tumors are five times less common than malignant tumors. With the introduction of newer and more sensitive diagnostic techniques [1] an increasing trend in the frequency of these lesions has emerged in comparison to old autopsy series where the overall prevalence was reported to be less than 1% [2, 3]. Benign esophageal masses can be classified by the cell of origin, by the wall layer, or by the radiographic appearance (Table 9.1). For the purpose of this chapter, we will focus on the most frequent lesions, i.e., leiomyoma, GIST, and extramucosal cysts. It is worthwhile to consider these conditions together because of their extramucosal origin in most patients, and because of the common diagnostic and therapeutic aspects. Most lesions are small and asymptomatic and therefore the real incidence in the general population may be underestimated. Usually, symptoms correlate with the site of the lesion. Intraluminal growths can present with mild dysphagia or obstruction, and extraluminal tumors may cause dyspnea due to airways compression. Chest pain and respiratory symptoms are often reported. Endoluminal bleeding from large ulcerated leiomyomas is rare and should rather alert toward the diagnosis of a gastrointestinal stromal tumor (GIST), a mesenchymal tumor distinct from leiomyoma that is more commonly found in the stomach and in the bowel. The diagnosis can be incidental during upper-GI endoscopy or computed tomography (CT) scan. For a more precise evaluation of the mass and the differential diagnosis with malignancies, endoscopic ultrasonography (EUS) and contrast CT-scan are mandatory [4]. The most common therapeutic option for esophageal leiomyoma is minimally invasive surgical enucleation through a laparoscopic or thoracoscopic

E. Asti (✉) • S. Siboni • L. Bonavina
Division of General Surgery, Department of Biomedical Sciences for Health,
University of Milano Medical School, IRCCS Policlinico San Donato, Milan, Italy
e-mail: emanuele.asti@grupposandonato.it

© Springer International Publishing AG, part of Springer Nature 2018
D. Oleynikov, P. M. Fisichella (eds.), *A Mastery Approach to Complex
Esophageal Diseases*, https://doi.org/10.1007/978-3-319-75795-7_9

Table 9.1 Synopsis for classification of benign esophageal tumors

Classification	Type	
By origin	Epithelial	Squamous cell papilloma Fibrovascular polyp Adenoma Inflammatory pseudotumor/polyp
	Nonepithelial	Leiomyoma Hemangioma Fibroma Neurofibroma Schwannoma Rhabdomyoma Lipoma Lymphangioma Hamartoma
	Heterotopic	Granular cell tumor Chondroma Osteochondroma Giant cell Amyloid Eosinophilic granuloma
By parietal layer	Mucosa	
	Submucosa	
	Muscolaris propria	
By radiologic aspect	Intramural-extramucosal	
	Intraluminal-mucosal	
	Extramural (cyst and duplication)	

approach. In some circumstances, leiomyomas at the gastroesophageal junctions may require a hybrid technique, such as a laparoscopic transgastric resection, or a full-thickness endoscopic enucleation.

Leiomyoma

The peak incidence is between the third and fifth decades, with a male to female ratio of 2. Leiomyoma accounts for over 50% of benign esophageal tumors: about 80% are intramural, arising from the muscularis propria in the lower and middle third of the esophagus. Gross pathological examination reveal a well encapsulated, round or oval-shaped mass, ranging from 0.5 to 5 cm in diameter. Microscopically, leiomyomas are composed of bundles of spindle cells with a very low rate of mitoses.

Occasionally, the mass can be significantly larger and becomes lobular or horseshoe shaped, and cause significant deformity of the esophageal lumen. The growth may be intra-luminal, extra-luminal, or horseshoe-shaped (Fig. 9.1). Immunohistochemistry is generally positive for smooth muscle actin and desmin (Table 9.2). Malignant degeneration is a very rare event.

Fig. 9.1 Typical
horseshoe leiomyoma

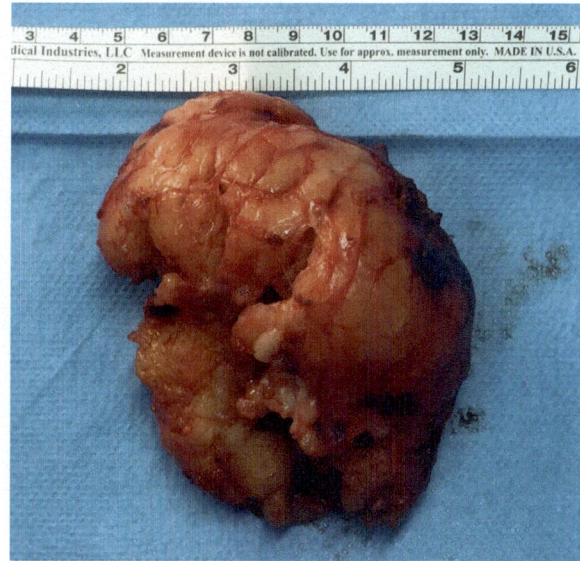

Table 9.2 Immunohistochemistry for differential diagnosis between leiomyoma and GIST

	Desmin	SMA (smooth muscle actin)	CD34	KIT (CD117)	S-100
Leiomyoma	+	+	–	–	Rare
GIST	Very rare	+ (30–40%)	+ (60–70%)	+	+ (5%)

Symptoms

Given the slow growth of the mass and the capacity of the esophagus to adapt and dilate, leiomyomas are generally asymptomatic. Dysphagia and pain are most commonly reported in symptomatic patients, especially when the tumor growth is intraluminal. Other symptoms are substernal discomfort, regurgitation, nausea and vomiting, cough, odynophagia, and heartburn [5]. Bleeding is rare and can result from ulceration of the overlying mucosa. In case of extramucosal growth, the mass can cause airway obstruction or compression on the vena cava [6].

Diagnosis

Half of the patients are asymptomatic and the majority of leiomyomas are found incidentally during upper gastrointestinal endoscopy or barium swallow study. In patients with symptoms and large tumors, an extensive workup is needed to plan the most appropriate treatment. The endoscopic findings consist of a protruding mass in the esophageal lumen with an intact, overlying mucosal layer (Fig. 9.2). In patients with previous bleeding, a central umbilication or ulceration can be found. Usually

Fig. 9.2 Bulging on the posterior esophageal wall just above the gastroesophageal junction with an intact overlying mucosa, suggesting leiomyoma

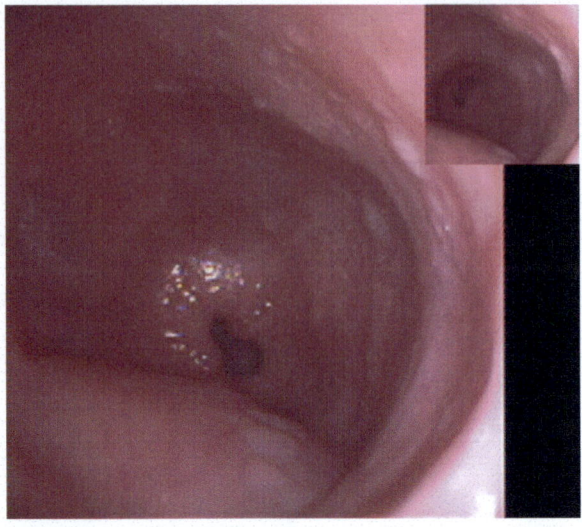

the mass does not prevent passage of the scope and peristalsis is not impaired. Several authors discourage endoscopic biopsies of the intact mucosa [1]. The radiological appearance of a leiomyoma on a barium contrast study is also typical: a round or oval mass with smooth mucosa (Fig. 9.3) [7], the presence of calcifications (non-specific), a sharp angle between the surrounding normal esophageal wall and the tumor, the obliteration of the lumen over the lesion, and the "forked stream sign" which consist in the splitting of the contrast to either side of the lesion. Computed tomography is needed to evaluate size and anatomic relationship of the tumor with the surrounding organs, particularly in case of large leiomyomas, and to exclude signs suggestive of malignancy (Fig. 9.4) [8]. Endoscopic ultrasonography (EUS) allows to better assess the size and the shape of the mass, and to identify the layer of the esophageal wall from which the mass arises. At EUS, the esophageal leiomyoma has a homogeneous and hypoechoic appearance [4], and no pathological mediastinal nodes are present. The differentiation between a leiomyoma and a GIST by EUS alone may prove difficult [4]. Hyperechogenicity, compared to the surrounding muscle layer, inhomogeneity of the mass, sometimes with the presence of spots and with a marginal halo, is more typical of GIST. A fine-needle aspiration biopsy can be performed in large tumors and when there is a suspicion of malignancy [9–12]. The diagnostic accuracy of EUS-guided FNA was found to range between 60% and 80%. Recent studies found a sensitivity of 96% and a specificity of 100% when the material was adequate for evaluation [8, 13].

Treatment

Small and asymptomatic masses can be managed conservatively, and an endoscopic ultrasound surveillance can be proposed. On the other hand, tumors greater than 3 cm, growth over time, mucosal ulceration, heterogeneous texture,

Fig. 9.3 Typical radiographic appearance of esophageal leiomyoma of the upper third of the thoracic esophagus

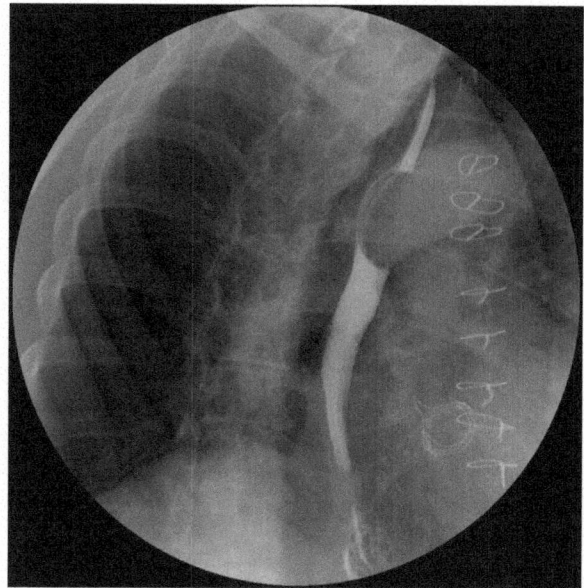

Fig. 9.4 CT thoracoabdominal scan showing a homogeneous circumferential thickening of the esophageal wall

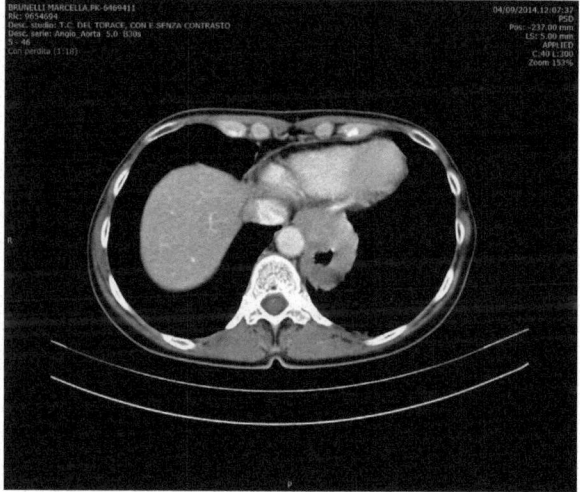

and surrounding lymph node enlargement are clear indications for resection (Fig. 9.5).

The open resection was the standard of care before the 90s, and the surgical approach consisted of right thoracotomy for upper two-third tumors, left thoracotomy for the lower third, and laparotomy for distal esophageal tumors [13]. Lately, minimally invasive techniques have been successfully applied in these patients and are now considered, the standard of care [14]. Given the benign nature of the tumor and the relative ease to dissect the mass from the muscle and mucosal layer, enucleation followed by muscle layer approximation is the treatment of choice [13].

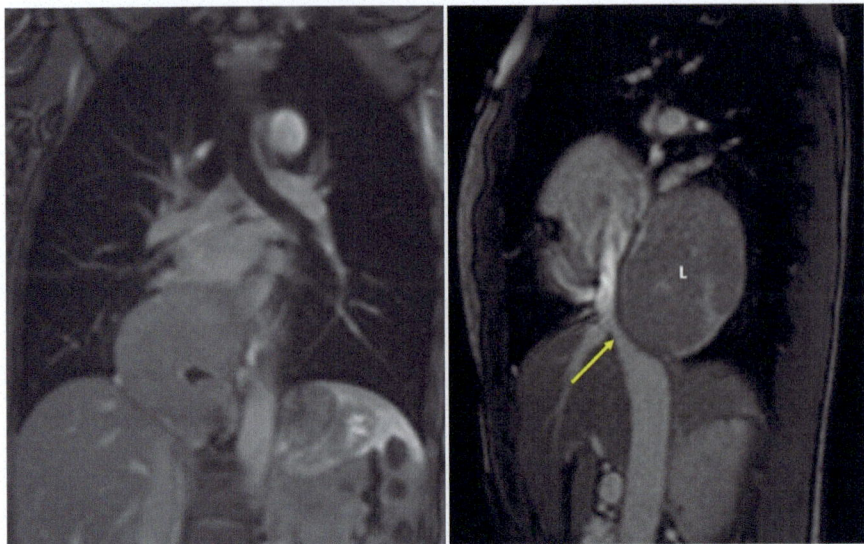

Fig. 9.5 Huge mediastinal leiomyoma causing compression of the cava vein

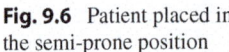

Fig. 9.6 Patient placed in the semi-prone position

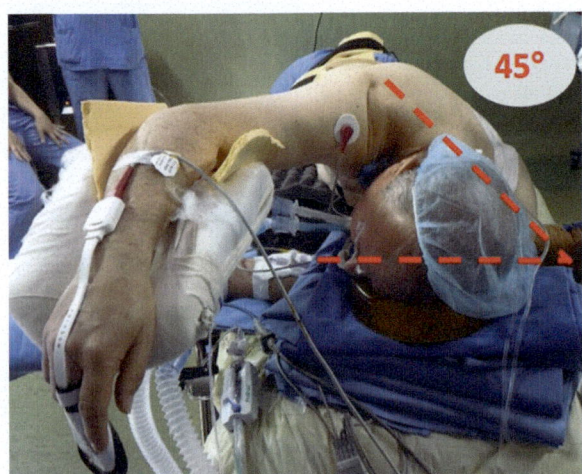

For the thoracoscopic approach, the patient is placed in the prone or semi-prone position (Fig. 9.6) [15]. Compared to the left lateral position, thoracoscopy in the prone position is associated with better ergonomics, a significant improvement of global oxygen delivery, and a reduction of the pulmonary shunt [16]. Regardless of the route of approach, enucleation of the leiomyoma requires an adequate mobilization of the esophagus above and below the site of the mass, opening of the mediastinal pleura, longitudinal splitting of the muscle layer overlying the mass, and gentle peeling away the muscle fibers, either bluntly or with of low-energy electrocoagulation. Care should be taken to preserve as much muscle layer as possible. A Penrose drain can be used for traction of the esophagus. A transfixed stitch can facilitate mobilization of the leiomyoma and identification of the cleavage plan from the mucosal layer [17]. Intraoperative endoscopy allows air inflation and transillumination, and may increase safety during the procedure [18]. Also, an endoscopic balloon inflated at the level of the leiomyoma can push the tumor outward and facilitate enucleation. Once the tumor is removed, the mucosa should be carefully inspected to ensure its integrity. In case a mucosal injury is recognized intraoperatively, it should be immediately repaired with interrupted absorbable stitches. Occurrence of a symptomatic pseudodiverticulum has been reported when leiomyoma enucleation is not followed by proper muscle approximation [13]. Access to upper esophageal leiomyomas may require preliminary division of the arch of the azygos vein using hem-o-lok clips or a vascular linear stapler. Nowadays, only in rare circumstances is a transthoracic or transhiatal videoassisted esophagectomy required (diffuse leiomyomatosis of the gastroesophageal junction, truly giant masses not eligible for enucleation, severe intraoperative complications. Recently, a robot-assisted resection of benign esophageal tumors has been described. This technology can provide better ergonomics and an easier dissection, but is more expensive [19, 20].

Laparoscopy is the preferred approach for tumors located at the gastroesophageal junction [21]. A standard 5-port access is required. The distal esophagus is encircled with a drain and pulled downwards. The most critical steps of the operation can be performed with endoscopic assistance. Care must be taken to avoid vagal nerve injuries during the dissection. An antireflux repair (Dor or Toupet fundoplication) after leiomyoma enucleation is recommended.

For giant (>10 cm) endophytic tumors prolapsing below the gastroesophageal junction, a laparoscopic transgastric approach may be the most appropriate option [22]. Endoscopic marking with endoclips of the distal tip of the tumor can facilitate the procedure. The anterior gastric wall is open longitudinally, the endoclips are easily identified, and the tumor mass is exteriorized. A linear endostapler can be applied at the base of the leiomyoma taking care not to cause deformity of the esophageal outlet. Endoscopic assistance can be helpful during this operative step. The anterior stomach wall is closed with a running suture or a linear endostapler, and a Dor fundoplication can be added to protect the wall and prevent gastroesophageal reflux.

Small esophytic tumors located on the anterior wall of the gastroesophageal junction or on the lesser curvature can be safely treated by a laparoscopic wedge resection. The key points to prevent anatomical deformity are the angle of insertion of the stapler and the use of multiple firings.

Gastrointestinal Stromal Tumor (GIST)

Esophageal GIST, with an annual incidence of approximately 7–19 cases per million, is the second most common mesenchymal tumor that originates from the interstitial cells of Cajal and is more commonly found in the stomach and small intestine. Only 5% of GIST are in the esophagus and more frequently at the gastro-esophageal junction. Microscopically, GIST present in three histologic subtypes: spindle cell

Table 9.3 Risk classification for GIST

Risk category	Tumor size (cm)	Mitotic count (per 50 HPFs)
Very low	<2	<5
Low	2–5	<5
Intermediate	<5	6–10
	5–10	<5
High	>5	>5
	>10	Any mitotic rate
	Any size	>10

type (most common), epithelioid type, and mixed spindle-epithelioid type. The malignant potential of GIST varies from virtually benign tumors to aggressive sarcomas. The 5-year overall survival rate after complete resection of GISTs is between 50% and 65%. The behavior of GIST is difficult to predict based on histopathology alone, and many factors like tumor size, mitotic rate, tumor location, kinase mutational status, and occurrence of tumor rupture play an important role as predictors of survival; tumor size and the proliferative index are the most widely accepted factors. The most used pathological classification, based on a NIH Consensus Conference, stratifies risk of an aggressive clinical course based on tumor size and mitotic count (Table 9.3) [23].

Symptoms and Diagnosis

Approximately 50% of patients are asymptomatic and the most common presentation is dysphagia or bleeding. The clinical presentation is dependent on the anatomic location of the tumor, the size, and its biological aggressiveness. The diagnostic workup should include a [18]FDG-PET that is highly sensitive and specific in detecting GIST and in evaluating the response to treatment.

Treatment

Complete surgical excision remains the cornerstone of management. Although there is no evidence suggesting that more extensive procedures prolong survival or delay recurrence, wedge or segmental resection are not applicable to esophageal tumors. Minimally invasive esophagectomy represents today the approach of choice, and the operation should follow the same oncological principles that are applied in patients with carcinoma.

Preoperative systemic therapy for GIST based on imatinib, a monoclonal antibody inhibiting the tyrosine-kinase c-kit protein, has led to a significant increase in median survival. Preoperative therapy can be used as a neoadjuvant regimen, for resectable tumor, or to downstage unresectable patients. Neoadjuvant therapy can lead to reduction in tumor size, making surgical resection safer and increasing the chance of getting negative margins. However, rapid reduction of the mass can cause necrosis followed by bleeding or perforation. For these reasons, the indications to imatinib treatment should be considered cautiously in these patients [24–26].

Extramucosal Cyst

Extramucosal cysts are congenital lesions of mixed embryogenesis. The origin is unknown and several theories have been proposed. Hutchison and Thomson hypothesized that at an initial stage of the development, a segment of endoderm is not correctly incorporated in the esophagus, thus forming a separate compartment with different histologic differentiation. According to the classification proposed by Arbona, cysts can be congenital (including bronchogenic, gastric, duplication or inclusion cysts), neuroenteric or acquired (retention cysts) [27].

Duplication cysts lie within the middle or the lower third of the esophagus; their wall is formed by two muscular layers and are covered by squamous or embryonic epithelium. Duplication cysts differ from inclusion cysts because the latter are not covered by muscle. The real incidence of extramucosal cysts is unknown. Autopsy studies hypothesize an incidence of 0.012%; about 40% of the cases occur in patients between 20 and 49 years of age [28].

Symptoms and Diagnosis

About one third of patients are asymptomatic at initial evaluation [29]. Among the symptomatic patients, there is a wide range of possible symptoms depending on the location, size and age of the patient. Respiratory symptoms, such as couch and wheezing are more common in children, while gastrointestinal symptoms, including gastroesophageal reflux, dysphagia, and epigastric pain occur more often in adults.

The diagnostic workup usually starts with an endoscopy or a barium swallow study, that look normal in the majority of the patients. Both CT-scan and EUS are recommended in these patients to assess the anatomy of the mass and the status of loco-regional nodes. Fine-needle aspiration cytology may be indicated in some circumstances to exclude malignancy [30].

Treatment

Asymptomatic patients may be followed over time with EUS or CT-scan. Indications for surgical treatment are the presence of dysphagia, respiratory symptoms, weight loss, increase in cyst size, and the suspicion of malignancy. The aspiration of the cyst content has been advocated as a minimally invasive technique for patients unfit for surgery. Laparoscopic or thoracoscopic resection remains the preferred treatment in expert hands [31]. The principles of the surgical approach are similar to that already described for leiomyoma, but stapling is usually required when dense adhesion to the esophageal wall are present.

Conclusions

Over the past few decades, the approach to leiomyoma, GIST and extramucosal cysts of the esophagus has changed significantly. The threshold for surgical indication is now lower due to the reduced morbidity and superior patient comfort provided by the minimally invasive techniques. Today, laparoscopy and thoracoscopy represent the initial approach even in large masses at unfavorable locations, and the conversion rate is low. It is important to tailor the approach according to the preoperative imaging and the site, size and shape of the mass. Endoscopic submucosal tunneling techniques for leiomyoma enucleation may play a major role in the future.

References

1. Rice TW. Benign esophageal tumors: esophagoscopy and endoscopic esophageal ultrasound. Semin Thorac Cardiovasc Surg. 2003;15:20–6.
2. Plachta A. Benign tumors of the esophagus. Review of literature and report of 99 cases. Am J Gastroenterol. 1962;38:639–52.
3. Attah EB, Hajdu SI. Benign and malignant tumors of the esophagus at autopsy. J Thorac Cardiovasc Surg. 1968;55(3):396–404.
4. Kim GH, Park do Y, Kim S, et al. Is it possible to differentiate gastric GISTs from gastric leiomyomas by EUS? World J Gastroenterol. 2009;15:3376–81.
5. Choong CK, Meyers BF. Benign esophageal tumors: introduction, incidence, and clinical features. Semin Thorac Cardiovasc Surg. 2003;15:3–8.
6. Lovece A, Milito P, Asti E, Bonavina L. Giant esophageal leiomyoma causing severe hypertension. BMJ Case Rep. 2016. https://doi.org/10.1136/bcr-2016-216837.
7. Glantz I, Grunebaum M. The radiological approach to leiomyoma of the esophagus with long-term follow-up. Clin Radiol. 1977;28:197–200.
8. Horton KM, Juluru K, Montgomery E, Fishman EK. Computed tomography imaging of gastrointestinal stromal tumors with pathology correlation. J Comput Assist Tomogr. 2004;28:811–7.
9. Caðlar E, Hatemi I, Atasoy D, et al. Concordance of endoscopic ultrasonography-guided fine needle aspiration diagnosis with the final diagnosis in subepithelial lesions. Clin Endosc. 2013;46:379–83.
10. Moon JS. Endoscopic ultrasound-guided fine needle aspiration in submucosal lesion. Clin Endosc. 2012;45:117–23.
11. Vander Noot MR 3rd, Eloubeidi MA, Chen VK, et al. Diagnosis of gastrointestinal tract lesions by endoscopic ultrasound-guided fine needle aspiration biopsy. Cancer. 2004;102:157–63.
12. Williams DB, Sahai AV, Aabakken L, et al. Endoscopic ultrasound guided fine needle aspiration biopsy: a large single centre experience. Gut. 1999;44:720–6.
13. Bonavina L, Segalin A, Rosati R, et al. Surgical therapy of esophageal leiomyoma. J Am Coll Surg. 1995;181:257–62.
14. Kent M, d'Amato T, Nordman C, et al. Minimally invasive resection of benign esophageal tumors. J Thorac Cardiovasc Surg. 2007;134:176–81.

15. Palanivelu C, Rangarajan M, Senthilkumar R, Velusany M. Combined thoracoscopic and endoscopic management of mid-esophageal benign lesions: use of the prone patient position. Surg Endosc. 2008;22:250–4.
16. Bonavina L, Laface L, Abate E, Punturieri M, Agosteo E, Nencioni M. Comparison of ventilation and cardiovascular parameters between prone thoracoscopic and Ivor Lewis esophagectomy. Updates Surg. 2012;64:81–5.
17. Lee LS, Singhal S, Brinster CJ, et al. Current management of esophageal leiomyoma. J Am Coll Surg. 2004;198:136–46.
18. Jeon HW, Choi MG, Lim CH, Park JK, Sung SW. Intraoperative esophagoscopy provides accuracy and safety in video-assisted thoracoscopic enucleation of benign esophageal submucosal tumors. Dis Esophagus. 2015;28:437–41.
19. Samphire J, Nafteux P, Luketich J. Minimally invasive techniques for resection of benign esophageal tumors. Semin Thorac Cardiovasc Surg. 2003;15:35–43.
20. Elli E, Espat NJ, Berger R, et al. Robotic-assisted thoracoscopic resection of esophageal leiomyoma. Surg Endosc. 2004;18:713–6.
21. Xu X, Chen K, Zhou W, Zhang R, Wang J, Wu D, Mou Y. Laparoscopic transgastric resection of gastric submucosal tumors located near the esophagogastric junction. J Gastrointest Surg. 2013;17:1570–5.
22. Song KY, Kim SN, Park CH. Tailored approach of laparoscopic wedge resection for treatment of submucosal tumors near the esophagogastric junction. Surg Endosc. 2007;21:2272–6.
23. Fletcher CD, Berman JJ, Corless C, et al. Diagnosis of gastrointestinal stromal tumors: a consensus approach. Hum Pathol. 2002;33:459–65.
24. Demetri GD, von Mehren M, Blanke CD, et al. Efficacy and safety of imatinib mesylate in advanced gastrointestinal stromal tumors. N Engl J Med. 2002;347:472–80.
25. Kawamura T, Asakawa T, Kaneshiro M, et al. A patient with esophageal GIST who developed pleuritis after imatinib treatment. Progress Dig Endosc. 2014;84:82–3.10.
26. Hecker A, Hecker B, Bassaly B, et al. Dramatic regression and bleeding of a duodenal GIST during preoperative imatinib therapy: case report and review. World J Surg Oncol. 2010;8:47.
27. Arbona JL, Fazzi GF, Mayoral J. Congenital esophageal cysts: case report and review of the literature. Am J Gastroenterol. 1984;79:177–82.
28. Whitaker J, Deffenbaugh L, Cooke A. Esophageal duplication cyst. Am J Gastroenterol. 1980;73:329–32.
29. Cioffi U, Bonavina L, De Simone M, et al. Presentation and surgical management of bronchogenic and esophageal duplication cysts in adults. Chest. 1998;113:1492–6.
30. Bondestam S, Salo JA, Salonen OLM, et al. Imaging of congenital esophageal cysts in adults. Gastrointest Radiol. 1990;15:279–81.
31. Noguchi R, Hashimoto T, Takeno S, et al. Laparoscopic resection of esophageal duplication cyst in an adult. Dis Esophagus. 2003;16:148–50.

Minimally Invasive Esophagectomy for Benign Disease

10

Chase Knickerbocker and Kfir Ben-David

History of Minimally Invasive Esophagectomy

The focus of this chapter is the application of minimally invasive esophagectomies (MIE) to benign disease processes. However, to understand this application one must first appreciate the history of MIE and the rigors to which is was subjected before it gained acceptance.

The Esophagus, a notoriously unforgiving organ, has been the subject of much debate and advances in operative technique in the last 100 years. The potential pitfalls of an open transhiatal esophagectomy are well known and include significant blind dissection that can result in hemorrhage, tracheal injury, and recurrent laryngeal nerve injury. As far back as the 1980s, pioneering researchers, including Kipfmuller, recognized that less invasive options were available. He and his colleagues went on to describe endoscopic esophageal dissections in animal models as early as 1989 [1].

As surgeon comfort with laparoscopic technique grew, the first case and small series reports of human patients undergoing endoscopically assisted esophagectomies for both malignant and benign esophageal disease surfaced [2]. In 1992 Cuschieri et al. described a successful series of five patients who underwent esophageal dissection via a right thoracoscopic approach. The survival of all five patients with reports of negligible blood loss in four of the five patients was the beginning of a revolution in the approach to esophageal surgery [3]. Alfred Cuschieri went on to explain that the procedures provided an unparalleled view of the dissection as well as detection of metastatic disease that was missed on pre-operative imaging. He also noted improvements in post-op recovery and equivalent lymphadenectomy as compared to open procedures [4]. Around the same time, Azagra, Collard, and several others showed success with laparoscopic esophageal dissection in patients with esophageal cancer as well as benign disease via thoracoscopy [5–8]. Although there

C. Knickerbocker, M.D., M.P.H. • K. Ben-David, M.D., F.A.C.S. (✉)
Mount Sinai Medical Center, Comprehensive Cancer Center, Miami Beach, FL, USA

© Springer International Publishing AG, part of Springer Nature 2018
D. Oleynikov, P. M. Fisichella (eds.), *A Mastery Approach to Complex Esophageal Diseases*, https://doi.org/10.1007/978-3-319-75795-7_10

were early detractors who did not fully support the new technique given the potential for pulmonary complications and prolonged operative times [9].

The basic approach involved a thoracoscopic esophageal dissection, abdominal esophagectomy, and cervical anastomosis. Basic principles championed by these early pioneers for a successful surgery included selection of patients with mobile esophageal tumors without local invasion, use of multiple viewing/working ports for appropriate visualization, double lumen endotracheal intubation for selective right lung collapse, the use of flexible gastroscopy to help with mobilization and retraction of the esophagus, high-quality illumination, and minimizing blood loss during dissection [7–9].

Even with the hybrid thoracoscopic technique well described, there was still no consensus that this approach should supplant the traditional open technique given a lack of clear survival and morbidity benefits [10, 11]. However, champions of the technique continued to persevere as there remained the matter of completing the abdominal portion of the dissection laparoscopically as well. DePaula and colleagues, who performed a series of 12 completely laparoscopic transhiatal esophagectomies for a combination of advanced achalasia and severe reflux stenosis, as well as oncologic indications, were the first to report on such an accomplishment. While there was one conversion to an open procedure, they reported no mortalities and established the legitimacy of a completely minimally invasive technique for esophagectomies [12]. Shortly thereafter Swanström and Hansen reported on a set of nine completely laparoscopic esophagectomies for benign strictures, Barrett's esophagus, and oncologic indications. All patients tolerated the initial surgeries well and one even underwent and thoracic anastomosis [13].

Despite these encouraging small case series, the reality remained that there was a dearth of evidence supporting MIE. The coming years would see larger publications regarding the efficacy of MIE. While there is little literature on the efficacy of MIE specifically for benign disease, several studies included patients treated for advanced achalasia, Barrett's esophagus, and refractory strictures. There appeared to be no lurking deleterious effects in these patient populations, and indeed they may fare better than cancer patients due to their overall health status. While evidence for MIE in benign disease is largely extrapolated from oncologic research, when performed in experienced hands, MIE procedures have the potential to decrease length of hospital stay and reduce the chance of postoperative pulmonary complications while offering similar rates of leaks [14–21]. It has even been shown to be safe and effective following previous gastric bypass surgery [22].

As we are discussing the evolution of the MIE, we must discuss potential advancements on the horizon. Robotics has, not without controversy, made an appearance in almost every surgical procedure including MIE. In small trials it appears as though patient undergoing robotic VATS are more susceptible to pulmonary complications, subjected to longer operative times, and potentially prone to greater blood loss. However, studies have noted that from an oncologic standpoint, there appears to be no substantial difference between the modalities [23–25]. Further exploration of this method is required especially with respect to operative length, cost benefit analysis, and reduction in morbidity associated with traditional thoracoscopy before a definitive opinion can be reached. At this time laparoscopic MIE remains the gold standard and as such the following discussion regarding operative technique will focus on this modality.

As with every surgical procedure, there are variations from institution to institution, but on the whole, minimally invasive esophagectomies fall within two broad categories. The two-site, Ivor-Lewis type dissection with thoracic anastomosis and the three-site McKeown type dissection with a cervical anastomosis. Both of these procedures are routinely performed at our institution and are described below.

Ivor-Lewis (Two-Site) Minimally Invasive Esophagectomy

The MIE variant of the Ivor-Lewis procedure utilizes a two-site approach while maintaining completely laparoscopic instrumentation. It can most easily be thought of as having distinct abdominal and thoracic portions. Presented here is the technique that we practice most routinely, including a side-to-side intra-thoracic stapled anastomosis.

First, the abdominal dissection is undertaken. The patient is placed in a supine position with a footboard to keep the patient in place, as steep reverse Trendelenberg positioning will be utilized during the case to facilitate the dissection. A double lumen endotracheal tube is also placed for selective collapse of the right lung for the thoracic dissection. The surgeon will be at the patient's right side for the procedure while the assistant will be on the patient's left.

The abdominal cavity is entered under direct visualization via a 5 mm trocar in the left subcostal region. After the initial trocar a 5 mm 30° angle scope is utilized to facilitate the placement of an additional three trocars under direct visualization: one 5 mm trocar in the supraumbilical region slightly to the left of the patient's midline; one 12 mm trocar in the right mid-abdominal region for the working right hand of the surgeon; one 12 mm trocar is placed in the right subcostal region at the midclavicular line for the working left hand of the surgeon; a final 5 mm subxiphoid incision is made to accommodate a liver retractor, lifting the left lobe of the liver exposing the gastroesophageal (GE) junction. The 5 mm ports in the umbilical and left subcostal areas will be for the assistant's laparoscope and retraction instrument, respectively.

At this time the abdomen is explored for metastatic disease and suspicious lesions are biopsied and sent to pathology for frozen evaluation. Assuming the pathology is benign, we are ready to begin the dissection.

The patient is placed in reverse Trendelenberg and the gastrohepatic ligament is taken down, exposing the GE junction. A window is created from the right crus to the angle of His forming a retrogastric space where a Penrose drain is placed and secured to help with mobilization of the GE junction. Taking great care not to enter the thoracic cavity, the left and right diaphragmatic crura are then widely dissected from the phrenoesophageal ligament. Patients with previous foregut surgery involving the distal esophagus and proximal stomach or who have undergone prior chemoradiation therapy can have scar tissue that makes the surgical dissection more difficult.

Next, the greater curvature of the stomach is taken down beginning with the origin of the gastroepiploic artery and vein and continuing to the angle of His. The right gastroepiploic arcade is preserved as future blood supply to the stomach. At times mobilizing the greater curvature of the stomach earlier may aid in defining the retrogastric plane. Connections between the stomach and the pancreas are then taken down and a limited mobilization of the first and second portions of the duodenum is performed. The left gastric artery and vein are dissected to their origins and division is performed with a vascular load stapler.

Creation of the gastric conduit begins at the lesser curvature of the stomach approximately 3 cm from the pylorus. From this point sequential firings of the 60 mm stapler are made in the direction of the angle of His. Care is taken to ensure the gastric conduit is approximately 6–7 cm in diameter. Lembert sutures, about four in total, are placed to reinforce the staple line junction sites and will also be used for retraction while working in the thoracic cavity. The gastric conduit is then reaffixed to the proximal stomach with silk sutures for mobilization. Finally, the distal aspect of the esophagus as the last remaining connection and is dissected free circumferentially.

The final part of the abdominal portion includes the placement of a jejunostomy tube 30–40 cm distal to the ligament of Treitz. A 16 French T-tube is utilized for this procedure at our institution. Of note, although we do not routinely perform pyloroplasties or Botox injections these do remain options for reducing postoperative gastric retention.

We now turn our attention to the thoracic portion of the procedure. The patient is placed in the left lateral decubitus position and the right lung is deflated. The surgeon will be posterior to the patient for the procedure. Initially the right chest cavity is entered via a 5 mm incision and trocar in the right subscapular region. A 5 mm 30° angled scope is again utilized and four additional trocars are placed under direct visualization: one 12 mm trocar is placed in the seventh intercostal space anterior to the mid axillary line for retracting the lung anteriorly during the dissection; one 5 mm port in the fifth intercostal space in line with the previously placed 12 mm trocar as the assistant's retraction port; one 5 mm trocar will be placed in the seventh intercostal space posterior to the mid axillary line as the surgeon's left hand working port; and one 12 mm trocar in the ninth or tenth intercostal space along the mid axillary line as the surgeon's right hand working port (Fig. 10.1).

The thoracic dissection begins with the opening of the posterior mediastinum at the level of the inferior pulmonary ligament. Circumferential dissection of the esophagus is completed with the aid of a Penrose drain and a blunt articulating dissector superiorly to a point above the azygos vein (Fig. 10.2). The azygos vein is then dissected and transected using a 60 mm vascular stapler via the right hand 12 mm port. The dissection of the esophagus continues to 3 cm above the azygos vein where the esophagus is divided using a stapler. The gastric conduit is then delivered into the right chest cavity.

It is now time to begin the anastomosis. Our preferred side to side alignment of the gastric conduit and esophagus is created and preserved with 2-0 braided, nonabsorbable stay sutures with long tails for future manipulation. A critical juncture is now reached where an esophagotomy must be made. A large bore nasogastric tube

Fig. 10.1 Thoracoscopic
port placement (Ivor-Lewis)

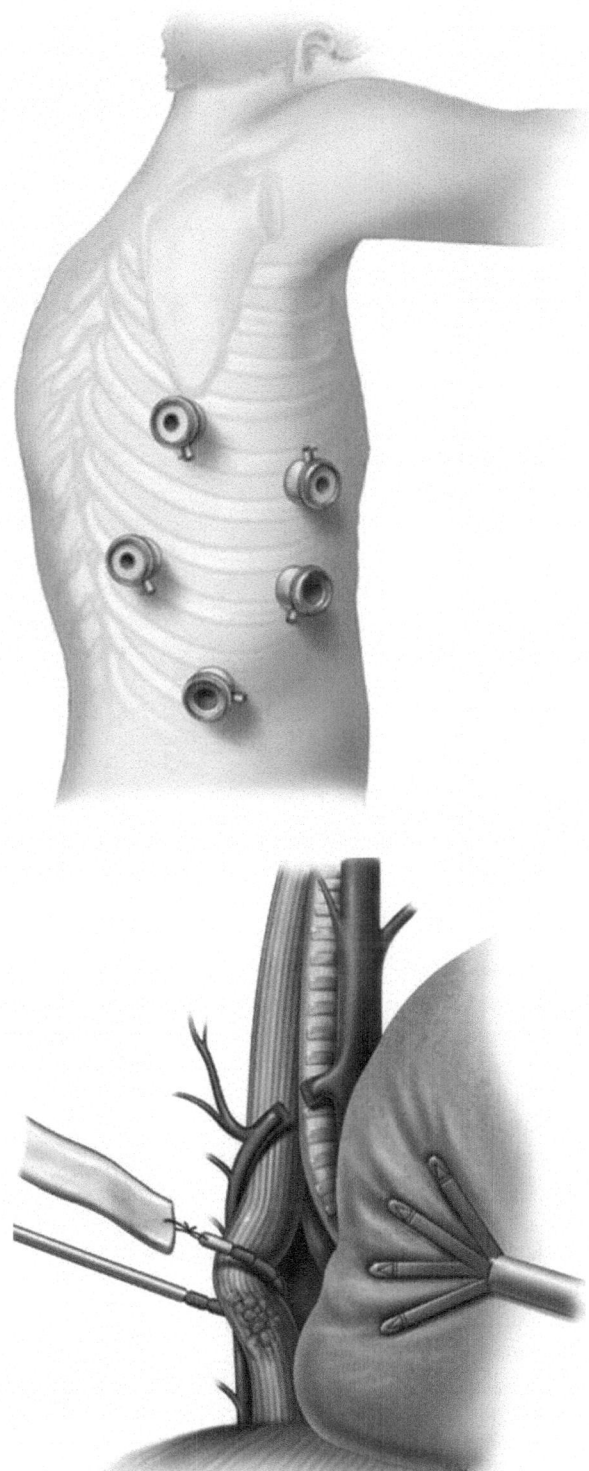

Fig. 10.2 Circumfrencial
esophageal dissection with
aid of Penrose drain

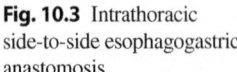

Fig. 10.3 Intrathoracic
side-to-side esophagogastric
anastomosis

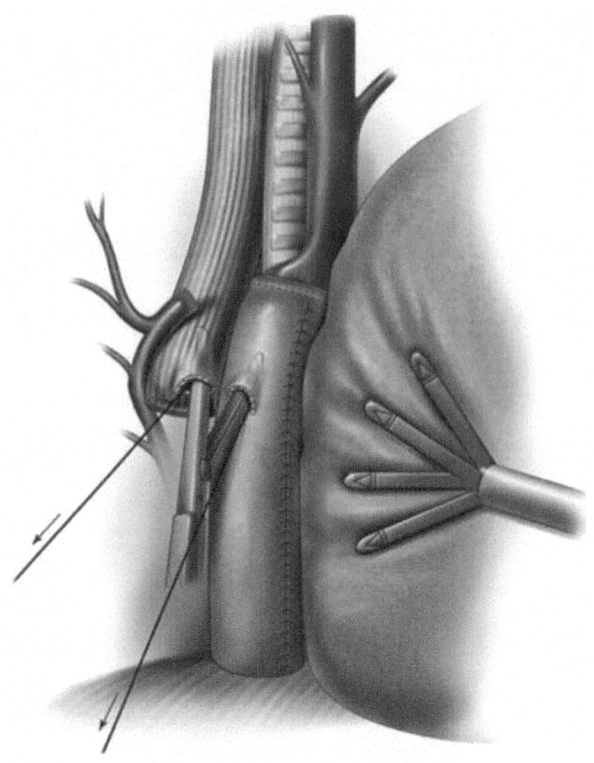

(NGT) or red rubber catheter is carefully advanced into the esophagus and used as a guide for creating the esophagotomy. A gastrotomy is then performed 8 cm proximal to the termination of the gastric conduit. A 60 mm stapler is inserted into the enterotomies and fired, creating a 6 cm esophagogastrostomy anastomosis (Fig. 10.3). Keep in mind, the stay sutures placed to hold the alignment of the esophagus and gastric tube may be used to help maintain alignment and provide traction while positioning the stapler. The anastomosis is now complete and the common opening of the prior esophagotomy and gastrotomy is approximated using an absorbable braided inner layer or a stapler followed by a non-absorbable outer layer. This anastomosis can also be performed using a circular end-to-end anastomosis.

With the completion of the anastomosis, an endoscopy is performed to visualize the patency of the conduit, inspect for bleeding, and most importantly the anastomosis is checked for leaks by insufflating air while submerging the anastomosis. With patency, hemostasis, and an airtight esophagogastrostomy achieved, the gastric conduit is secured to the diaphragm with two 2-0 silk sutures. The conduit may also be secured to the pleura if necessary.

Removal the specimen is done through a 3 cm thoracotomy at the fifth intercostal space that requires no rib spreading. A 24 French thoracotomy tube is then placed in the posterior mediastinum to facilitate drainage and help with leak detection without the aid of suction. The NGT is left in place [26].

McKeown (Three-Site) Minimally Invasive Esophagectomy

Although there are similarities between this technique and the MIE Ivor-Lewis approach, the most glaring dissimilarity is the addition of a cervical dissection and anastomosis. Although it is beyond the scope of this chapter to provide an in depth debate on which method of surgery is better or preferred in a particular patient, this method is preferred by our institution.

To begin, the patient is intubated with a double lumen endotracheal tube and an 18 gauge nasogastric tube is placed. The patient is initially placed in the left lateral decubitus position. The right lung in deflated and the initial 5 mm trocar is placed just inferior to the right scapula and a 5 mm 30° scope is used for the duration of the thoracoscopic dissection. Insufflation is achieved in the right chest cavity to 8 mm Hg of carbon dioxide. Three additional trocars are then placed: One 5 mm trocar directly posterior to the initial trocar in the posterior axillary line at the seventh intercostal space as the left hand working port for the surgeon; one 5 mm trocar in the posterior axillary line at the tenth intercostal space for the right working hand of the surgeon; and one 5 mm trocar placed anteriorly in the seventh intercostal space and will be utilized for retraction of the lung via a fan retractor (Fig. 10.4).

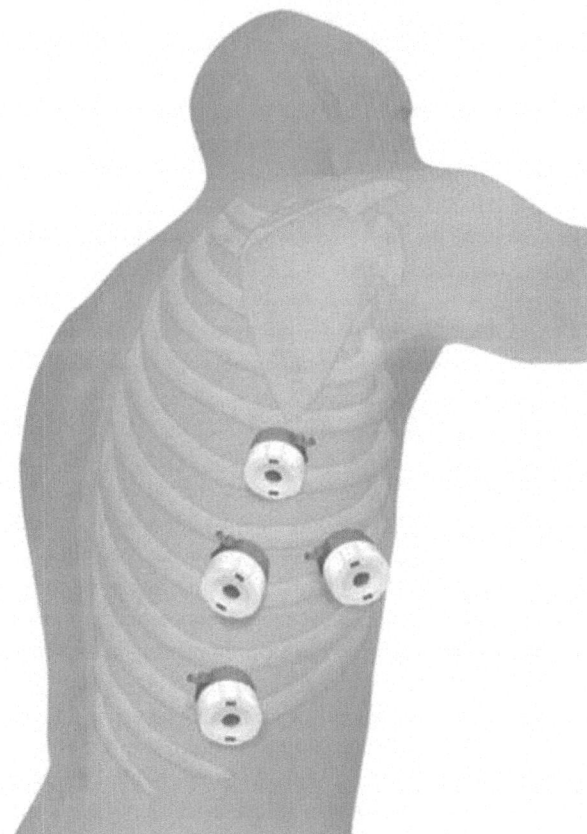

Fig. 10.4 Thoracoscopic port placement (McKeown type)

At this point and dissection begins with anterior retraction of the right lung and division of the inferior pulmonary ligament. Dissection of the esophagus can then begin utilizing a combination of bipolar cautery, a blunt articulating dissector, and Penrose drain secured loosely around the esophagus with an endo-loop tie. This allows the drain to slide up and down the esophagus to facilitate dissection and retraction. Dissection begins at the GE junction and proceeds in a cephalad direction taking care not to enter the left chest cavity or the abdomen. The azygos vein will be encountered and is divided using a 45 or 60 mm vascular load stapler. If the thoracic duct is noted during the dissection, it is also ligated to help prevent unintentional damage and chyle leaks. After ligation of the azygos vein and dissection off the esophagus, mobilization of the esophagus off the trachea continues up through the level of the thoracic inlet. The cervical dissection is essentially completed via the thoracoscopic approach. It is felt that this provides lower chance of damage to the recurrent laryngeal nerve as it is done under direct camera visualization and within the plane between the trachea and the esophagus. With the cervical and thoracic esophageal dissections completed, the Penrose drain will be directed up to the cervical esophagus and kept in place for now. Closing this portion of the procedure involves placing a 24 French Blake drain in the posterior mediastinum that exits through the inferior 12 mm trocar site. The remaining sites are closed in the usual fashion and the drain is secured.

At this time, attention is turned to the cervical area. The patient is repositioned in the supine position with the left arm tucked and head rotated for left neck exposure. A footboard is used to help secure the patient, as steep reverse Trendelenburg will be used for the abdominal dissection. After prepping of the neck, chest, and abdomen, a 6 cm incision is made at the anterior border of the sternocleidomastoid muscle (SCM). The SCM is retracted laterally and the omohyoid muscle is divided. Approaching the prevertebral fascial plane requires ligation of bridging veins as well as lateral retraction of the carotid artery and jugular vein. After entering the prevertebral fascial plane, the Penrose should be visible and secured with a Kelly clamp. Given the thoracoscopic dissection of the cervical esophagus, this portion if the procedure should be relatively quick.

Attention is now turned to the abdomen for dissection of the distal esophagus and stomach. A 5 mm trocar is placed under direct visualization in the left subcostal area as the assistants port and three additional trocars are placed: one 5 mm trocar 2 cm to the left and above the umbilicus for the 30° angled scope; one 12 mm trocar at the same level as the camera port and just lateral to the rectus muscle on the right side as the surgeon's right hand working port; and one final 12 mm trocar is placed 6 cm superior and lateral to the existing 12 mm port as the surgeon's left hand working port.

The patient is placed in steep Trendelenburg and a 5 mm incision is made just inferior and to the left of the xiphoid process to facilitate placement of a Nathanson liver retractor. At this point there are nine steps to the abdominal dissection that must be followed. First, dissecting and securing the GE junction with a Penrose is accomplished by dissection the tissue of the right crus of the diaphragm and carefully passing a grasper from right to left behind the stomach and just inferior to the left crus of the diaphragm to create a retrogastric conduit. The Penrose can be secured with an endo-loop. The second portion involves mobilization of the upper aspect of the greater curvature of the stomach by entering the lesser sac about half way up the greater curvature and, with the use of a tissue-sealing device, dividing the gastrocolic omentum and short gastric vessels until the left crus and Penrose drain are identified. Care is taken with this step to preserve the right gastroepiploic vessels. The third step involves the lower part of the greater curvature, which is taken down in the same manner mentioned above. The stomach is also mobilized off the pancreas till the gastroduodenal artery is visualized.

For the fourth step, attention is turned to the duodenum. The first and second sections are mobilized from the superior aspect by the surgeon till the bile duct is reached. A full Kocher maneuver is usually not necessary but may be utilized in cases where more conduit mobility is needed. The fifth step involves transecting the right gastric artery about 4 cm proximal to the pylorus. At this time the left gastric artery and vein are transected as the sixth step. This requires careful dissection down to the base of the celiac trunk. This allows for a thorough lymphadenectomy along the vessels in oncologic operative settings. The dissection is then continued up to the GE junction.

The seventh step is particularly important and involves crafting the gastric conduit. This begins along the lesser curvature of the stomach 4 cm proximal to the pylorus and will require 5–6 serial firings of a 60 mm endo-stapler with 2.5–3 mm staples. The first firing sets the appropriate width for the gastric conduit, 6–7 cm in diameter. At this point the NGT should also be retracted so it is at the GE junction, well out of the line of fire. Serial firings of the stapler are carried out along the body and fundus of the stomach. Withhold the last firing till each of the staple lines is reinforced with a single inverting 2-0 silk suture. The tails should be left long as they will play in important roll in mobilizing the stomach.

The eighth step involves freeing the GE junction by widely excising the phreno-esophageal ligament and continuing the dissection up the esophagus till it meets the thoracic portion. Again to help with mobilization, the gastric conduit is secured to the remnant stomach with simple interrupted 2-0 silk sutures. The ninth and final step involves transferring the stomach/gastric conduit up to the neck. This takes a team approach, the assistant will, with the help of the Penrose left around the cervical esophagus, deliver the esophagus, GE junction, and gastric conduit through the cervical incision while the surgeon preserves the orientation of the gastric conduit, preventing twisting.

Attention is now turned back to the neck for the cervical esophagogastrostomy anastomosis. This initially involves delivery of the gastric conduit and esophagus from the cervical incision and opposing the posterior portion of the stomach and the medial aspect of the esophagus. Electro cautery is used to enter the distal aspect of the esophagus that will be preserved as well as the gastric conduit about 8 cm from where it terminates. The nasogastric tube is pulled out from the esophageal opening and a 6 cm stapler with the anvil in the esophagus and the staple load in the gastric tube (Fig. 10.5). After firing, the nasogastric tube is placed into the gastric tube through the anastomosis and a stapler is used to close the common opening. This staple line is reinforced with a running 3-0 PDS suture and the crotch is secured

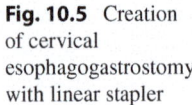

Fig. 10.5 Creation of cervical esophagogastrostomy with linear stapler

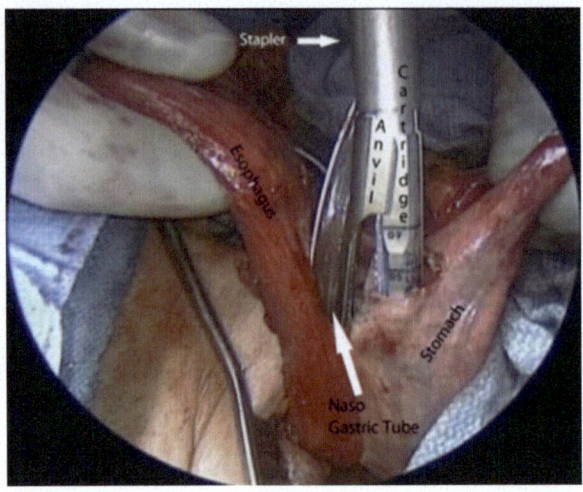

with two simple 3-0 silk sutures. The anastomosis is delivered back into the cervical incision and a 7 French drain (not under suction) is placed along side the anastomosis and exits posterior to the SCM. The gastric conduit is then secured to the diaphragm with 2 2-0 silk sutures and a 16 French jejunal feeding tube is inserted and the port sites are closed in the usual fashion [27].

The postoperative management of an esophagectomy patient is an exercise in patience. Overall, the goal is the ensure that the anastomosis is acceptable for use before removing the drains and allowing the patient unrestricted by mouth intake and this takes at least several days of inpatient care. This section will discuss the postoperative management of esophagectomy patients including our institutions typical course and possible variations to consider for your practice and will be broken down by the goals associated with each postoperative day.

In the immediate postoperative setting, postoperative day 0, patients have several milestones that must be met. All patients are expected to be up and sitting in a chair the evening of surgery, incentive spirometer use is mandated ten times per hour while awake, and their indwelling urinary catheter removed at midnight in anticipation of voiding trial in the morning. Ambulation at this point is encouraged and at the very least the patient will be performing assisted transfers from the bed to the chair. Patients are kept strictly nothing by mouth and drain output is monitored. It is important to note that the drains are left to gravity drainage as it is felt that the added suction of bulbs and/or wall suction will contribute to anastomotic breakdown and increase leak rates.

Postoperative day 1 the patient remains strictly nothing by mouth and feeds are started per the jejunostomy at 10 mL per hour and increased by a rate of 10 mL every 12 h as tolerated by the patient to a goal determined by the unit dietitian. Drain output is monitored and the patient begins to ambulate several times per day. Pain control and incentive spirometer use is key at this time to help prevent postoperative pneumonias, the most likely cause of morbidity following minimally invasive esophagectomy, seen in 28.5% of patients [28]. Hence, the nasogastric tube is typically removed on postoperative day 3 or 4 since there is a high association with nasogastric tube and aspiration pneumonia.

At the point the patient will be focusing on ambulation, physical therapy, incentive spirometry, and receiving jejunal feeds until the anastomosis is evaluated. This is typically performed on postoperative day 5 at our institution via a fluoroscopic contrast swallow esophagram looking for extravasation of contrast and collection within the drainage catheters. Following a successful swallow study, the patient is trialed on a clear liquid diet under direct observation of the surgeon with a colorful clear liquid, typically cranberry juice. This particular test is looking for both juice in the drains as well as signs of aspiration which is not uncommon given the literature notes most, if not all patients have some degree of impaired swallowing following esophagectomy, especially with a cervical dissection [29].

Assuming the patient passes all of the benchmarks, they are ready for discharge on a full liquid diet with advancement back to a regular diet over the following several weeks. The level of impaired swallowing in the immediate postoperative setting largely determines the initial diet as thinner liquids can pose a problem for some patients. In the unfortunate event a leak is noted, the patient will remain nothing by mouth with drains in place for two more weeks before reattempting a fluoroscopic swallow evaluation. These patients are difficult to manage as they are prone to septic events and the drains are an absolute necessity for source control. Often times, patients can still be discharged and a follow-up swallow study can be done as an outpatient.

Variations to this postoperative theme include the used of endoscopy to check the anastomosis, which is advocated by some surgeons as safe while also giving them the opportunity to check for ischemia or questionable areas of the anastomosis under direct visualization. It has been the experience of our team that this places unnecessary stress on the anastomosis and there is frequently a small degree of ischemia noted at the anastomosis without any clinical consequences and may result in an unnecessary workup or delay in returning the patient to a diet. The jejunostomy tube will remain in place until the patient is tolerating enough calories by mouth and can be removed in the office during a postoperative visit.

In summary, MIE has become a well-accepted modality for the treatment of esophageal disease, both benign and malignant. However, there is a steep learning curve and advanced training in the appropriate laparoscopic skills is necessary for a surgeon to successfully perform these operations. Perhaps more importantly, it is not a solitary surgeon that will make or break a successful MIE program, but an entire team of appropriately trained OR staff, technicians, nurses, dietitians, speech and language pathologists, and physical therapists. The total team approach is essential to getting the patients safely through surgery and on the post-operative road to recovery.

References

1. KipfmuLler K, et al. Endoscopic microsurgical dissection of the esophagus. Surg Endosc. 1989;3(2):63–9. https://doi.org/10.1007/bf00590902.
2. Dallemagne B, et al. Case report: subtotal oesophagectomy by thoracoscopy and laparoscopy. Minim Invasive Ther. 1992;1(2):183–5. https://doi.org/10.3109/13645709209152942.
3. Cuschieri A, et al. Endoscopic oesophagectomy through a right thoracoscopic approach. J R Coll Surg Edinb. 1992;37:7–11.
4. Cuschieri A. Endoscopic subtotal oesophagectomy for cancer using the right thoracoscopic approach. Surg Oncol. 1993;2:3–11. https://doi.org/10.1016/0960-7404(93)90052-z.
5. Azagra JS, et al. Thoracoscopy in oesophagectomy for oesophageal cancer. Br J Surg. 1993;80(3):320–1. https://doi.org/10.1002/bjs.1800800317.
6. Collard JM, et al. En bloc and standard esophagectomies by thoracoscopy. Ann Thorac Surg. 1993;56(3):675–9. https://doi.org/10.1016/0003-4975(93)90949-i.
7. Gossot D, et al. Thoracoscopic esophagectomy: technique and initial results. Ann Thorac Surg. 1993;56(3):667–70. https://doi.org/10.1016/0003-4975(93)90947-g.
8. Cuschieri A. Right subtotal thoracoscopic oesophagectomy with lymphadenectomy. Oper Man Endosc Surg. 1994;2:103–20. https://doi.org/10.1007/978-3-662-01566-7_4.
9. Mcanena OJ, et al. Right thoracoscopically assisted oesophagectomy for cancer. Br J Surg. 1994;81(2):236–8. https://doi.org/10.1002/bjs.1800810225.
10. Gossot D, et al. Can the morbidity of esophagectomy be reduced by the thoracoscopic approach? Surg Endosc. 1995;9(10):1113–5. https://doi.org/10.1007/bf00188998.
11. Law S, et al. Thoracoscopic esophagectomy for esophageal cancer. Surgery. 1997;122(1):8–14. https://doi.org/10.1016/s0039-6060(97)90257-9.
12. DePaula AL, et al. Laparoscopic transhiatal esophagectomy with esophagogastroplasty. Surg Laparosc Endosc. 1995;5(1):1–5.
13. Swanstrom LL. Laparoscopic total esophagectomy. Arch Surg. 1997;132(9):943. https://doi.org/10.1001/archsurg.1997.01430330009001.
14. Luketich JD, et al. Minimally invasive esophagectomy. Trans Meet Am Surg Assoc. 2003;121:179–88. https://doi.org/10.1097/01.sla.0000089858.40725.68.
15. Luketich JD, et al. Minimally invasive esophagectomy. Ann Surg. 2015;261(4):702–7. https://doi.org/10.1097/sla.0000000000000993.
16. Ben-David K, et al. Decreasing morbidity and mortality in 100 consecutive minimally invasive esophagectomies. Surg Endosc. 2011;26(1):162–7. https://doi.org/10.1007/s00464-011-1846-3.
17. Ben-David K, et al. Minimally invasive esophagectomy is safe and effective following neoadjuvant chemoradiation therapy. Ann Surg Oncol. 2011;18(12):3324–9. https://doi.org/10.1245/s10434-011-1702-7.
18. Sgourakis G, et al. Minimally invasive versus open esophagectomy: meta-analysis of outcomes. Dig Dis Sci. 2010;55(11):3031–40. https://doi.org/10.1007/s10620-010-1153-1.
19. Lv L, et al. Minimally invasive esophagectomy versus open esophagectomy for esophageal cancer: a meta-analysis. Onco Targets Ther. 2016;9:6751–62. https://doi.org/10.2147/ott.s112105.
20. Nguyen NT, et al. Thoracoscopic and laparoscopic esophagectomy for benign and malignant disease: lessons learned from 46 consecutive procedures. J Am Coll Surg. 2003;197(6):902–13. https://doi.org/10.1016/j.jamcollsurg.2003.07.005.
21. Kim T, et al. Review of minimally invasive esophagectomy and current controversies. Gastroenterol Res Pract. 2012;2012:1–7. https://doi.org/10.1155/2012/683213.
22. Rossidis G, et al. Minimally invasive esophagectomy is safe in patients with previous gastric bypass. Surg Obes Relat Dis. 2014;10(1):95–100. https://doi.org/10.1016/j.soard.2013.03.015.
23. Van Hillegersberg R, et al. First experience with robot-assisted thoracoscopic esophagolymphadenectomy for esophageal cancer. Surg Endosc Other Interv Tech. 2006;20(9):1435–9. https://doi.org/10.1007/s00464-005-0674-8.

24. Okusanya LT, et al. Robotic assisted minimally invasive esophagectomy (RAMIE): the University of Pittsburgh Medical Center initial experience. Asvide. 2017;4:342. https://doi.org/10.21037/asvide.2017.342.
25. Boone J, et al. Robot-assisted thoracoscopic oesophagectomy for cancer. Br J Surg. 2009;96(8):878–86. https://doi.org/10.1002/bjs.6647.
26. Ben-David K, et al. Technique of minimally invasive ivor lewis esophagogastrectomy with intrathoracic stapled side-to-side anastomosis. J Gastrointest Surg. 2010;14(10):1613–8. https://doi.org/10.1007/s11605-010-1244-5.
27. Hochwald SN, Ben-David K. Minimally invasive esophagectomy with cervical esophagogastric anastomosis. J Gastrointest Surg. 2012;16(9):1775–81. https://doi.org/10.1007/s11605-012-1895-5.
28. Atkins BZ, et al. Reducing hospital morbidity and mortality following esophagectomy. Ann Thorac Surg. 2004;78(4):1170–6. https://doi.org/10.1016/j.athoracsur.2004.02.034.
29. Atkins BZ, et al. Analysis of respiratory complications after minimally invasive esophagectomy: preliminary observation of persistent aspiration risk. Dysphagia. 2006;22(1):49–54. https://doi.org/10.1007/s00455-006-9042-7.

Barrett Esophagus

11

Vic Velanovich

Introduction

Barrett esophagus is a change in the normal squamous epithelium of the esophagus to specialized columnar-lined epithelium first recognized by Norman Barrett [1]. Barrett esophagus is associated with gastroesophageal reflux disease (GERD) and is a risk factor for esophageal adenocarcinoma. It has been an area of intense interest due to the increased incidence of esophageal adenocarcinoma and being a potential target for prevention. It is incumbent on practitioners who treat patients with esophageal disease to understand Barrett esophagus and its management.

Pathogenesis

The precise sequence of molecular events that lead to the development of Barrett's esophagus have not been completely elucidated. It is hypothesized that the development of Barrett's metaplasia is a protective mechanism to chronic inflammation and tissue injury related to acid and bile exposure. There are numerous theories as to how the normal squamous esophageal epithelium transforms into Barrett metaplasia [2]. Kapoor, et al. [2] nicely summarize these theories: (1) migration of cells from the gastric epithelium, which, at this point, does not appear to be a major factor in the development of Barrett metaplasia. (2) The transdifferentiation of native squamous epithelium. In this theory, embryonic esophageal columnar epithelium differentiates into squamous epithelium due to activation of prosquamous and inactivation of procolumnar homeobox genes. Due to chronic acid and bile exposure, reverse activation occurs leading to development of columnar epithelium. (3) Reparative emergence of submucosal glanular stem cells. The neck region of the

V. Velanovich, M.D.
Division of General Surgery, University of South Florida, Tampa, FL, USA
e-mail: vvelanov@health.usf.edu

© Springer International Publishing AG, part of Springer Nature 2018
D. Oleynikov, P. M. Fisichella (eds.), *A Mastery Approach to Complex Esophageal Diseases*, https://doi.org/10.1007/978-3-319-75795-7_11

esophageal submucosal glands contain stem cells. It is theorizes that these stem cells differentiate into columnar cells as a response to chronic inflammatory refluxate. (4) Transcommitment of resident squamous stem cells. Stems cells in the interpapillary zone of the basal cell layer of the squamous epithelium undergo abnormal differentiation into columnar epithelium. (5) Colonization by circulating bone marrow derived stem cells. In this theory, circulating pluripotent adult progenitor cells from the bone marrow infiltrate and regenerate damaged squamous epithelium and developed into columnar metaplasia. (6) Residual embryonic cells at the transitional zone between the squamous and columnar epithelium at the Z-line. In this theory, it is activation of persistent, but quiescent, embryonic stems cells at the transition between the esophageal squamous and gastric columnar epithelium which differentiate into Barrett metaplasia rather than the normal adult cell populations transdifferentiating or transcommiting. (7) Luminal unfolding of esophageal retention cysts. This theory rests on resident esophageal retention cysts becoming disrupted due to chronic reflux, thus allowing there columnar cells to spread over the esophageal mucosal surface. In all of these theories, the unified underlying driving mechanism of injury is chronic acid and duodenogastroesophageal reflux. It is the combined exposure to both acid and bile than is seen in the most severe cases of complicated Barrett's esophagus.

Once Barrett metaplasia is established, there are additional genetic alternations which are required to progress to adenocarcinoma. Morphologically, Barrett esophagus progresses in a stepwise fashion from metaplasia to low-grade dysplasia to high-grade dysplasia to intramucosal adenocarcinoma to invasive adenocarcinoma. This morphological change is driven by genomic, transcriptomic and epigenetic changes [3]. In the acid environment, GPX3 is downregulated and NOX5 is upregulated leading to blockage of the normal esophageal protective mechanism. NOX5, in particular, leads to over production of reactive oxygen species in the cells causing mutations in several genes. The TP53 mutation leads to prevention of normal apoptosis of damaged cells. In conjugation with NOX5 mediate hypermethylation of CDKN2A-p16INK4A promoter, proliferation is enhanced. In a potentially separate pathway, CDH1 downregulation also leads to abnormal proliferation through overexpression of the MYC and CCND1 genes [3]. Nevertheless, despite these advanced in our knowledge of the molecular events leading to progression to adenocarcinoma, it is also clear that our knowledge is incomplete and further work needed.

Epidemiology and Risk Factors

Prevalence

It is difficult to know the true prevalence of Barrett esophagus due to the fact that many individuals are asymptomatic and, therefore, will never be identified. The best estimate of the population prevalence of Barrett esophagus is 1.6% of the general population [4]. It is believed that the prevalence of Barrett esophagus has increased, paralleling to the increase in esophageal adenocarcinoma [5]. A Swedish study demonstrated that symptomatic individuals had a prevalence of Barrett esophagus of 2.3%, compared to 1.4% in asymptomatic individuals [6].

Incidence

The incidence of Barrett esophagus is even more difficult to estimate than prevalence. Most studies have relied on follow-up of patients who have manifestations of GERD or calculations based on population estimates. The Kalixanda study [7] of a general Swedish population initially found endoscopic or histologic diagnosis of GERD and nonerosive reflux disease (NERD), of these patients 9.7% of patients with NERD progressed to erosive esophagitis, and 1.8% to Barrett esophagus. In patients initially with erosive esophagitis, 13.3% progress to a more severe grade and 8.9% to Barrett esophagus [7]. The overall incidence of Barrett esophagus was 9.9 per 1000 person years [7].

The incidence of Barrett esophagus appears to be increasing. Coleman, et al. [8] found that the annual incidence from 2002 to 2005 was 62.0 per 100,000 persons per year, showing an increase 159% compared to 1993–1997. This incidence increased most markedly in patients <60 years, especially in men <40 years.

Risk Factors

Risk factors for the development of Barrett esophagus include GERD, obesity, male gender, Caucasian ethnicity, and increasing age. Smoking may increase the risk of Barrett esophagus, whereas Helicobacter pylori infection, and specific "healthy" dietary factors may lower the risk [9]. Nelsen [10] compared 50 Barrett esophagus patients to matched controls with computed tomography scan to determine gastroesophageal junction fat area, visceral fat area, and abdominal circumference. Visceral and gastroesophageal junction fat were significantly greater among patients with Barrett esophagus (odds ratio [OR] 6.0; 95% CI 1.3–27.7) independent of body mass index.

Tobacco smoking increases the risk of Barrett esophagus. Subjects with Barrett esophagus were significantly more likely to have ever smoked cigarettes than the population-based controls (OR 1.67; 95% CI 1.04–2.67) or GERD controls (OR 1.61; 95% CI 1.33–1.96) [11]. Increasing pack-year history of smoking increased the risk of Barrett esophagus. There was synergy of smoking with GERD with the attributable proportion of disease among individuals who ever smoked and had heartburn or regurgitation was 0.39 (95% CI 0.25–0.52) [11].

Diets high in fiber and "good" fats reduce the risk of Barrett esophagus. Higher intake of omega-3 fatty acids (OR 0.46; 95% CI 0.22–0.97), polyunsaturated fat, total fiber (OR 0.34; 95% CI 0.15–0.76), and fiber from fruits and vegetables (OR 0.47; 95% CI 0.25–0.88) were associated with a lower risk. Higher meat intakes were associated with a lower risk of "long-segment" Barrett esophagus (OR 0.25; 95% CI 0.09–0.72). Conversely, higher trans-fat intakes were associated with increased risk of Barrett esophagus (OR 1.11; 95% CI 1.03–1.21). Total fat intake, barbecued foods, and fiber intake from sources other than fruits and vegetables were not associated with Barrett esophagus [12].

Some social issues may be associated with Barrett esophagus. German patients with Barrett esophagus and adenocarcinoma tend to have higher incomes [13]. Barrett esophagus appears less prevalent among persons of Asian, Caribbean, African, Middle Eastern, and South American origin [14]. African Americans with Barrett esophagus are less likely than whites to have long- segment disease (12% vs. 26%) and dysplasia (0% vs. 7%) [15].

Progression to Adenocarcinoma

At present, our best way to estimate the progression of Barrett esophagus is primarily histologic grade. Non-dysplastic epithelium progresses at a rate of 3.86 per 1000 persons per year [16], low-grade dysplasia at 7.66 per 1000 persons per year [17], and high-grade dysplasia at 146 per 1000 persons per year [17]. The progression rate of high-grade dysplasia appears to be lower than the occult carcinoma rate discovered in esophagectomy specimens of high-grade dysplasia of 30% [18]. Age, male gender, and Barrett metaplasia length only modestly increase the risk of progression to carcinoma [19, 20].

Current smoking, former smoking, and >40 years of smoking increased the risk of progression to HGD and esophageal adenocarcinoma; whereas current alcohol use did not, but former alcohol use did [21].

Multiplex familial kindreds, defined as families with three or more members with Barrett esophagus or esophageal adenocarcinoma, have a younger median age at diagnosis of esophageal adenocarcinoma (57 vs. 62 years old) and a lower body mass index [22]. It is estimated that 6.2% of patients with Barrett esophagus, 9.5% of patients with esophageal adenocarcinoma, and 9.5% of patients with gastroesophageal junction adenocarcinoma have a first or second degree relative with familial Barrett esophagus [23].

Diagnosis

Surprisingly, the definition of Barrett esophagus is not completely settled. The proximal displacement of the squamocolumnar junction is essential for the diagnosis, but there are different methodologies used to identify the gastroesophageal junction [24]. Identification of the "palisade" of vessels in the lower esophagus with identification of the top of the gastric folds and the diaphragmatic pinch, constitute the essential endoscopic landmarks. Endoscopically, Barrett esophagus appears as a salmon colored epithelium extending proximal from the gastroesophageal junction (Fig. 11.1a). In cases where the border between the abnormal Barrett epithelium and normal squamous epithelium is difficult to distinguish, narrow band imaging can bring out the distinction (Fig. 11.1b). Barrett esophagus length should be classified

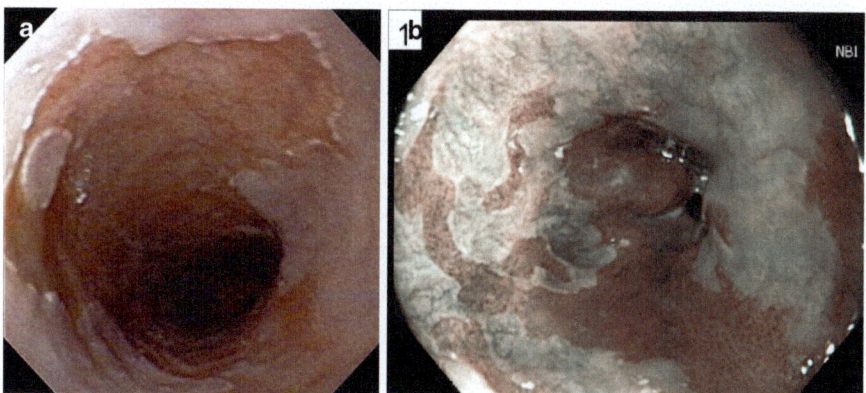

Fig. 11.1 (**a**) Endoscopic view of Barrett esophagus using white light. (**b**) Endoscopic view of Barrett esophagus using narrow band imaging

using the Prague system based on circumferential and total length of metaplasia. For example, if 2 cm of esophagus is circumferentially involved with Barrett metaplasia and there is an additional 2 cm tongue of Barrett metaplasia extending from this, this would be classified as C2M4 [25].

Pathologic diagnosis is not based on world-wide uniformed criteria. In Europe, the histologic diagnosis is based on detection of any type of glandular mucosa with goblet cells, while in the United States, intestinal metaplasia with goblet cells is the most widely used histologic criteria [26]. The key basis for this recommendation is the increased incidence of esophageal adenocarcinoma among patients with endoscopic Barrett esophagus with intestinal metaplasia compared with patients who have endoscopic Barrett esophagus without intestinal metaplasia [26]. An international consensus group recommended that all pathology reports should state the presence or absence of goblet cells in the diagnosis of Barrett's metaplasia [27].

Grading of dysplasia is a pathologic determination. There are several possible interpretations from the pathologist: (1) negative for dysplasia; (2) positive for dysplasia, either LGD or HGD; or (3) indefinite for dysplasia [28]. However, the interobserver variability is problematic [29]. Therefore, expert review or a review by a panel of experts is essential to ensure the most accurate diagnosis.

Management of Barrett Esophagus

Prevention

There are two types of prevention associated with Barrett esophagus: primary prevention of Barrett esophagus and prevention of progression of Barrett esophagus to esophageal adenocarcinoma.

Chemoprevention is related to either prevention of esophageal acid exposure or modulation of proinflammatory mechanisms. Chemoprevention with proton pump inhibitors (PPIs), statins, and aspirin or nonsteroidal anti-inflammatory agents is based on epidemiologic evidence [9]. Patients who consume aspirin had a reduced prevalence of Barrett esophagus (OR 0.56; 95% CI 0.39–0.80) [30]. Regular use of statins was associated with a significantly lower incidence of esophageal cancer in patients with Barrett esophagus (OR 0.45; 95% CI 0.24–0.84). The combination of statins with aspirin further reduced the risk (OR 0.31; 95% CI 0.04–0.69) [31]. Nevertheless, without randomized, prospective data, it is not recommended that patients with Barrett esophagus without other indications for aspirin or statins should be administered these medications solely for the prevention of progression to esophageal adenocarcinoma.

Screening

In 2016, the American College of Gastroenterologist have published new guidelines in the diagnosis and management of Barrett esophagus [32]. With respect to screening, they do not recommend screening endoscopy for either the general population or women with GERD. In men with a >5 year history of GERD and having ≥2 risks factors (age >50 years, male sex, white race, increased body mass index, and intra-abdominal distribution of fat, current or former smoker and family history of Barrett esophagus or esophageal adenocarcinoma), screening may be appropriate [32]. If screening is done and no Barrett esophagus is found, no further screening is necessary or desirable [32].

Treatment

Acid suppression without surveillance is based on the premise that screening has not been shown to improve mortality from adenocarcinoma or to be cost effective [33]. Barbiere and Lyratzapoulos [34] have questioned a variety of assumptions made for these recommendations. Therefore, the recommendation for acid suppression without surveillance should be made with caution and thorough patient counseling.

Acid suppression with surveillance identifies early-stage esophageal adenocarcinoma. Because there are no reliable data on the duration of PPI treatment, most practitioners will keep patients on PPI therapy indefinitely. Wong, et al. [35] showed that 80% of esophageal adenocarcinomas found in patients undergoing surveillance were stage I cancers, compared with only 6.5% in patients who were not in the surveillance program ($P < 0.001$). These data imply that cancers are indeed found earlier when patients are undergoing surveillance. Although the optimal frequency of surveillance has not been determined, most authorities recommend surveillance at intervals of 3–5 years for patients with nondysplastic metaplasia, 6–12 months for LGD, and every 3 months for HGD in patients not receiving invasive therapy [36].

Antireflux surgery in experienced hands usually in the form of some type of fundoplication, eliminates acid, and bile reflux in more than 90% of patients with

Barrett esophagus [37]. Factors to consider in the choice between medical and surgical management include reflux-related symptoms, comorbidities, patient choice, adverse effects of medications, and individual surgeon skill. Prospective studies [38, 39] have demonstrated regression of Barrett esophagus in patients who have undergone laparoscopic Nissen fundoplication. A meta- analysis of antireflux surgery compared with medical treatment in GERD patients with Barrett esophagus demonstrated a pooled estimate of 15.4% of patients who have undergone antireflux surgery will have regression of Barrett esophagus compared with 1.9% of medically managed patients [40]. Nevertheless, the evidence that antireflux surgery lowers the risk for progression to adenocarcinoma is mixed [41–43]. Therefore, although antireflux surgery can successfully treat reflux-related symptoms in patients with Barrett esophagus, caution should be used when discussing its role in Barrett regression or protection against progression to adenocarcinoma.

Although different types of endoscopic ablative therapies are available, the AGA [44], the National Institute for Health and Clinical Excellence in the United Kingdom [45], and the Society of American Gastrointestinal and Endoscopic Surgeons [46] have recommended ablation only with radiofrequency ablation (RFA), photodynamic therapy (PDT), or endoscopic mucosal resection (EMR) for patients with Barrett esophagus with HGD.

PDT consists of injecting a light-sensitizing drug into the patient, then exposing the portion of the esophagus to light of a specific wavelength which would then lead to metaplasia and dysplasia cell death [47]. However, eradication of both nondysplastic metaplasia and HGD and prevention of adenocarcinoma has been variable [48, 49], with issues involving "buried glands." In addition, especially with long segments of Barrett esophagus, stricture formation was up to 40% [50], with these strictures being difficult to dilate. For these reasons, PDT, although still considered an acceptable treatment, has lost favor.

RFA applies bipolar electrical energy to the mucosal surfaces at energy levels of 10 Joules for 1 s. With this technique, the mucosa is ablated to the submucosal level [51, 52]. Generally, within several weeks to a few months postablation, the exposed submucosal esophageal surface resurfaces with a "neosquamous" epithelium (Fig. 11.2). Endoscopic RFA is an effective means of eliminating Barrett metaplasia [48]. Using standardized follow-up protocols, complete ablation can be achieved in over 90% of patients [53, 54]. A meta-analysis and systematic review of the incidence of adenocarcinoma in patients with Barrett esophagus treated with ablative therapies compared with historical controls showed a reduction in carcinoma progression in nondysplastic metaplasia, in LGD, and especially in HGD [55]. A landmark randomized trial has demonstrated superiority of endoscopic RFA compared with sham procedure in reducing the progression to adenocarcinoma of HGD [56]. RFA has been shown to be durable, complete eradication of intestinal metaplasia 91%, 96% for HGD, and 100% for LGD, with no disease progression occurring in 1 per 73 patient years of follow-up and progression to adenocarcinoma occurring in 1 per 181 patient years [57]. However, ablation of longer segments of Barrett esophagus is associated with a higher rate of both persistent and recurrent metaplasia compared with segments shorter than 3 cm in length [53]. A recent randomized

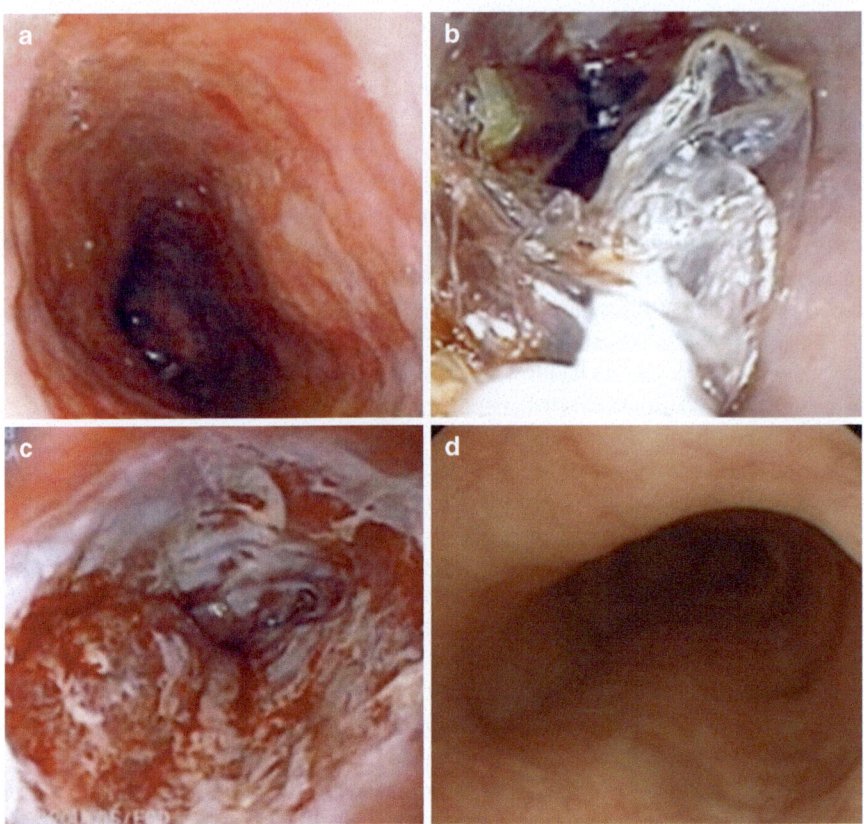

Fig. 11.2 Steps in radiofrequency ablation of Barrett esophagus. (**a**) Identification of proximal extent of Barrett metaplasia. (**b**) Deflated ablation balloon after ablation completed. (**c**) Immediate ulcer caused by ablation. (**d**) Normal squamous epithelium after completion of healing

controlled trial comparing surveillance to RFA in patients with low grade dysplasia demonstrated at 3 years of follow-up a reduction in the progression to adenocarcinoma from 8.8% in the surveillance group to 1.5% in the RFA treated group [58].

Cryoablation involves endoscopically directed spray of liquid nitrogen at −196° C directly onto the Barrett epithelium [59]. Complete eradication of Barrett HGD has been reported in 68–97% of patients [60, 61], of intestinal metaplasia occurs in 57% [61], and intramucosal adenocarcinoma in 80% [60]. Nevertheless, cryoablation is not as well studied as RFA and is yet to be determined if it is an alternative or complementary treatment.

EMR is a valuable technique to remove nodular Barrett esophagus with HGD (Fig. 11.3). The technique is most useful when either a visible nodule is present or only a short segment of Barrett epithelium is seen. One particular advantage of EMR is that it provides tissue pathologic review. EMR can also be used for Tis or T1a esophageal adenocarcinoma. However, an endoscopic ultrasound examination is essential to ensure that the submucosa is not involved [48]. EMR can be

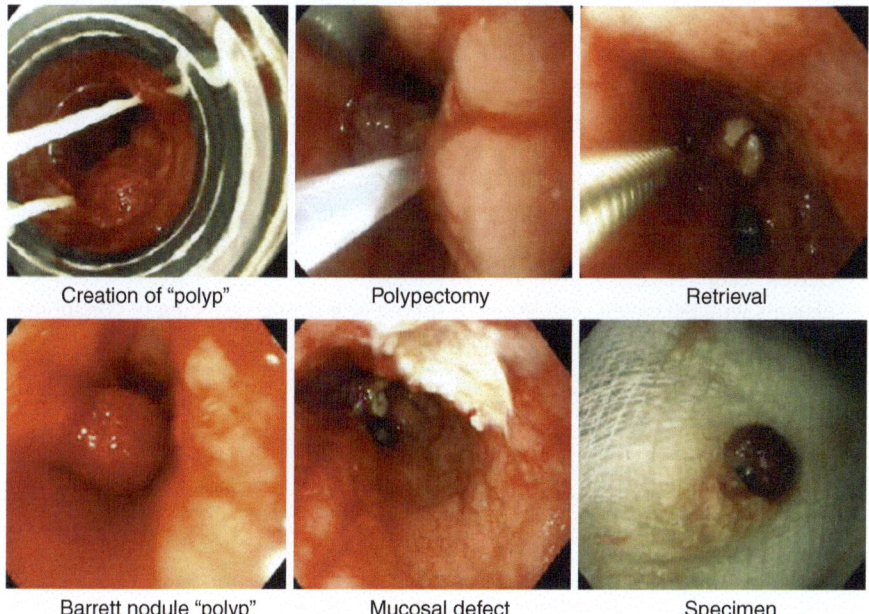

Creation of "polyp"   Polypectomy   Retrieval

Barrett nodule "polyp"   Mucosal defect   Specimen

Fig. 11.3 Steps in EMR of a Barrett's nodule

combined with RFA to allow for resection of the nodular component of Barrett HGD with ablation of the remaining field of flat Barrett metaplasia [62].

Endoscopic RFA has been used in conjunction with antireflux operations. Firstly, RFA in patient with pre-existing antireflux operation was associated with no change in reflux symptoms after ablation [63]. Secondly, combining endoscopic ablation with an antireflux operation reduces the overall number of procedures that a patient must undergo [64]. Lastly, the presence of a fundoplication reduces the recurrence or persistence of Barrett esophagus [65]. This is consistent with the findings of Krishnan and colleagues [66] who also have shown that recurrence after RFA was related to uncontrolled reflux.

Esophagectomy was considered a reasonable approach to patients with HGD. The rationale was that 20–40% of patients with HGD on biopsy will actually harbor an early-stage adenocarcinoma [67, 68]. Although esophagectomy can be performed with very low mortality, morbidity is still high. Even if the operation is accomplished without morbidity, the detrimental effects on quality of life are significant [69]. Therefore, esophagectomy should be reserved only for patients for whom ablation has not led to durable eradication of HGD or if suspicion for carcinoma is high. When esophagectomy is performed for Barrett esophagus, vagus-preserving esophagectomy should be considered [70]. The addition of a fundoplication after an esophagectomy has been shown to decrease the incidence of recurrent Barrett esophagus in the remnant esophagus from 18% to 6% [71]. The type of fundoplication used involves created gastric flaps from the apex of the gastric remnant, then creating the esophagogastrostomy inferior to the flaps, then bringing the flaps around to create the fundoplication.

Conclusions

Although there are many unanswered questions with Barrett esophagus, we can safely say that the incidence in on the rise, chemoprevention strategies for the prevention of Barrett metaplasia and its progression to adenocarcinoma may be on the offing, surveillance should be considered for all patients who are discovered to have Barrett esophagus, RFA is the treatment of choice for those with high-grade dysplasia and strongly considered in those with low-grade dysplasia, EMR should be the treatment of choice for patients with nodular high-grade Barrett esophagus, and, finally, vagal-sparing esophagectomy reserved for patients with persistent high-grade dysplasia or a strong suspicion of carcinoma, with consideration of a concomitant fundoplication.

References

1. Barrett NR. Chronic peptic ulcer of the oesophagus and 'oesophagitis. Br J Surg. 1950;38:175–82.
2. Kapoor H, Agrawal DA, Mittal SK. Barrett's esophagus: recent insights into pathogenesis and cellular ontogeny. Transl Res. 2015;166:28–40.
3. Kalataskaya I. Overview of major molecular alternations during progression from Barrett's esophagus to esophageal adenocarcinoma. Ann N Y Acad Sci. 2016;1381:74–91.
4. Wang KK, Practice Parameters SRE. Committee of the American College of Gastroenterology. Updated guidelines 2008 for the diagnosis, surveillance and therapy of Barrett's esophagus. Am J Gastroenterol. 2008;103:788–97.
5. Spechler SJ. Clinical practice. Barrett's esophagus. N Engl J Med. 2002;346:836–42.
6. Ronkainen J, Aro P, Storskrubb T, et al. Prevalence of Barrett's esophagus in the general population: an endoscopic study. Gastroenterology. 2005;129:1825–31.
7. Ronkainen J, Talley NJ, Storskrubb T, et al. Erosive esophagitis is a risk factor for Barrett's esophagus: a community-based endoscopic follow-up study. Am J Gastroenterol. 2011;106:1946–52.
8. Coleman HG, Bhat S, Murray LJ, et al. Increasing incidence of Barrett's oesophagus: a population-based study. Eur J Epidemiol. 2011;26:739–45.
9. Winberg H, Lindblad M, Lagergren J, Dahlstrand H. Risk factors and chemoprevention in Barrett's esophagus—an update. Scand J Gastroenterol. 2012;47:397–406.
10. Nelsen EM, Kirihara Y, Takahashi N, et al. Distribution of body fat and its influence on esophageal inflammation and dysplasia in patients with Barrett's esophagus. Clin Gastroenterol Hepatol. 2012;10:728–34.
11. Cook MB, Shaheen NJ, Anderson LA, et al. Cigarette smoking increases the risk of Barrett's esophagus: an analysis of the Barrett's and Esophageal Adenocarcinoma Consortium. Gastroenterology. 2012;142:744–53.
12. Kubo A, Block G, Queensberry CP Jr, et al. Effects of dietary fiber, fats, and meat intakes on the risk of Barrett's esophagus. Nutr Cancer. 2009;61:607–16.
13. Gao L, Weck MN, Rothenbacher D, Brenner H. Body mass index, chronic atrophic gastritis and heartburn: a population-based study among 8936 older adults from Germany. Aliment Pharmacol Ther. 2010;32:296–302.
14. Falk GW, Jacobson BC, Riddell RH, et al. Barrett's esophagus: prevalence-incidence and etiology-origins. Ann N Y Acad Sci. 2011;1232:1–17.
15. Khoury JE, Chisholm S, Jamal MM, et al. African Americans with Barrett's esophagus are less likely to have dysplasia at biopsy. Dig Dis Sci. 2012;57:419–23.

16. Sharma P, Falk GW, Weston AP, et al. Dysplasia and cancer in a large multicenter cohort of patients with Barrett's esophagus. Clin Gastroenterol Hepatol. 2006;4:566–72.
17. Verbeek RE, van Oijen MG, ten Kate FJ, et al. Surveillance and follow-up strategies in patients with high-grade dysplasia in Barrett's esophagus: a Dutch population-based study. Am J Gastroenterol. 2012;107:534–42.
18. Buttar NS, Wang KK, Sebo TJ, et al. Extent of high-grade dysplasia in Barrett's esophagus correlates with risk of adenocarcinoma. Gastroenterology. 2001;120:1630–9.
19. Prasad GA, Bansal A, Sharma P, Wang KK. Predictors of progression in Barrett's esophagus: current knowledge and future directions. Am J Gastroenterol. 2010;105:1490–502.
20. Coleman HG, Bhat S, Johnston BT, et al. Tobacco smoking increases the risk of high-grade dysplasia and cancer among patients with Barrett's esophagus. Gastroenterology. 2012;142:233–40.
21. de Jorge PJF, Steyerberg EW, Kuipers EJ, et al. Risk factors for the development of esophageal adenocarcinoma in Barrett's esophagus. Am J Gastroenterol. 2006;101:1421–9.
22. Chak A, Chen Y, Vengoechea J, et al. Variation in age at cancer diagnosis in familial versus nonfamlial Barrett's esophagus. Cancer Epidemiol Biomarkers Prev. 2012;21:376–83.
23. Chak A, Ochs-Balon A, Falk G, et al. Familiality in Barrett's esophagus adenocarcinoma of the esophagus and adenocarcinoma of the gastroesophageal junction. Cancer Epidemiol Biomarkers Prev. 2006;15:1668–773.
24. Boyce HW. Endoscopic definitions of esophagogastric junction regional anatomy. Gastrointest Endosc. 2000;51:586–92.
25. Alvarez-Herrero L, Curvers WL, van Vilsteren FG, et al. Validation of the Prague C and M classification of Barrett's esophagus in clinical practice. Endoscopy. 2013;45:876–82.
26. Naini BV, Souza RF, Odze RD. Barrett's esophagus: a comprehensive and contemporary review for pathologists. Am J Surg Pathol. 2016;40:e45–66.
27. Bennett C, Moayyedi P, Corley DA, et al. BOB CAT: a large-scale review and Delphi consensus for management of Barrett's esophagus with no dysplasia, indefinite for, or low-grade dysplasia. Am J Gastroenterol. 2015;110:662–82.
28. Goldblum JR. Controversies in the diagnosis of Barrett esophagus and Barrett-related dysplasia: one pathologist's perspective. Arch Pathol Lab Med. 2010;134:1479–84.
29. Downs-Kelly E, Mendelin JE, Bennett AE, et al. Poor interobserver agreement in the distribution of high-grade dysplasia and adenocarcinoma in pretreatment Barrett's esophagus biopsies. Am J Gastroenterol. 2008;103:2333–40.
30. Omer ZB, Ananthakrishnan AN, Nattinger KJ, et al. Aspirin protects against Barrett's esophagus in a multivariate logistic regression analysis. Clin Gastroenterol Hepatol. 2012;10:722–7.
31. Beales IL, Vardi I, Dearman L. Regular statin and aspirin use in patients with Barrett's oesophagus is associated with a reduced incidence of oesophageal adenocarcinoma. Eur J Gastroenterol Hepatol. 2012;24:917–23.
32. Shaheen NJ, Falk GW, Iyer PG, Gerson LB. ACG clinical guidelines: diagnosis and management of Barrett's esophagus. Am J Gastroenterol. 2016;111:30–50.
33. Garside R, Pitt M, Somerville M, et al. Surveillance of Barrett's oesophagus: exploring the uncertainty through systematic review, expert workshop and economic modeling. Health Technol Assess. 2006;10:1–142.
34. Barbiere JM, Lyratzopoulos G. Cost-effectiveness of endoscopic screening followed by surveillance for Barrett's esophagus: a review. Gastroenterology. 2009;137:1869–76.
35. Wong T, Tian J, Nager AB. Barrett's surveillance identifies patients with early esophageal adenocarcinoma. Am J Med. 2010;123:462–7.
36. Maes S, Sharma P, Bisschops R. Review: surveillance of patients with Barrett oesophagus. Best Pract Res Clin Gastroenterol. 2016;30:901–12.
37. Oelschlager BK, Barreca M, Chang L, et al. Clinical and pathologic response of Barrett's esophagus to laparoscopic antireflux surgery. Ann Surg. 2003;238:458–64.
38. Biertho L, Dallemagne B, Dewandre J-M, et al. Laparoscopic treatment of Barrett's esophagus: long-term results. Surg Endosc. 2007;21:11–5.

39. Knight BC, Devitt PG, Watson DI, et al. Long-term efficacy of laparoscopic antireflux surgery on regression of Barrett's esophagus using Bravo wireless pH monitoring: a prospective clinical cohort study. Ann Surg. 2017;266:1000–5.
40. Chang EY, Morris CD, Seltman AK, et al. The effect of antireflux surgery on esophageal carcinogenesis in patients with Barrett's esophagus: a systematic review. Ann Surg. 2007;246:11–21.
41. Gurski RR, Peters JH, Hagen JA, et al. Barrett's esophagus can and does regress after antireflux surgery: a study of prevalence and predictive features. J Am Coll Surg. 2003;196:706–12.
42. Bowers SP, Mattar SG, Smith CD, et al. Clinical and histologic follow-up after antireflux surgery for Barrett's esophagus. J Gastrointest Surg. 2002;6:532–8.
43. Lagergren J, Ye W, Lagergren P, Lu Y. The risk of esophageal adenocarcinoma after antireflux surgery. Gastroenterology. 2010;138:1297–301.
44. AGA Institute Medical Position Position Panel. American Gastroenterological Association medical position statement on the management of Barrett's esophagus. Gastroenterology. 2011;140:1084–91.
45. National Institute for Health and Clinical Excellence. CG 106 Barrett's oesophagus—ablative therapy: NICE guideline. http://guidance.nice.org.uk/CG106S. Accessed 14 Oct 2012.
46. Stefandis D, Hope WW, Kohn GP, et al. Guidelines for surgical treatment of gastroesophageal reflux disease. Surg Endosc. 2010;24:2647–69.
47. Wang KK, Song LMWK, Buttar N, et al. Barrett's esophagus after photodynamic therapy: risk of cancer development during long-term follow-up. Gastroenterology. 2004;126(suppl 2):A50.
48. Menon D, Stafinski T, Wu H, et al. Endoscopic treatments for Barrett's esophagus: a systematic review of safety and effectiveness compared to esophagectomy. BMC Gastroenterol. 2010;10:111.
49. Overholt BF, Wang KK, Burdick JS, et al. Five-year efficacy and safety of photodynamic therapy with Photofrin in Barrett's high-grade dysplasia. Gastrointest Endosc. 2007;66:460–8.
50. Prasad GA, Wang KK, Buttar NS, et al. Predictors of stricture formation after photodynamic therapy for high grade dysplasia in Barrett's esophagus. Gastrointest Endosc. 2007;65:60–6.
51. Dunkin BJ, Martinez J, Bejarano PA, et al. Thin-layer ablation of human esophageal epithelium using a bipolar radiofrequency balloon device (BARRx). Surg Endosc. 2006;20:125–30.
52. Smith CD, Bejarano PA, Melvin WS, et al. Endoscopic ablation of intestinal metaplasia containing high-grade dysplasia in esophagectomy patients using a balloon-based ablation system. Surg Endosc. 2007;21:560–9.
53. Velanovich V. Endoscopic endoluminal radiofrequency ablation of Barrett's esophagus: initial results and lessons learned. Surg Endosc. 2009;23:2175–80.
54. Wani S, Puli SR, Shaheen NJ, et al. Esophageal adenocarcinoma in Barrett's esophagus after endoscopic ablative therapy: a meta-analysis and systematic review. Am J Gastroenterol. 2009;104:502–13.
55. Li YM, Li L, Yu CH, et al. A systematic review and meta-analysis of the treatment for Barrett's esophagus. Dig Dis Sci. 2008;53:2837–46.
56. Shaheen NJ, Sharma P, Overholt BF, et al. Radiofrequency ablation in Barrett's esophagus with dysplasia. N Engl J Med. 2009;360:2277–88.
57. Shaheen NJ, Overholt BF, Sampliner RE, et al. Durability of radiofrequency ablation in Barrett's esophagus with dysplasia. Gastroenterology. 2011;141:460–8.
58. Phoa KN, van Vilsteren FG, Weusten BLA, et al. Radiofrequency ablation vs. endoscopic surveillance for patients with Barrett esophagus and low-grade dysplasia: a randomized clinical trial. JAMA. 2014;311:1209–17.
59. Johnston MH, Eastone JA, Horwhat JD, et al. Cryoablation of Barrett's esophagus: a pilot study. Gastrointest Endosc. 2005;62:842–8.
60. Dumot JA, Vargo JJ II, Falk GW, et al. An open-label prospective trial of cryospray ablation for Barrett's esophagus high-grade dysplasia and early esophageal cancer in high-risk patients. Gastrointest Endosc. 2009;70:635–44.
61. Shaheen NJ, Greenwald BD, Peery AF, et al. Safety and efficacy of endoscopic spray cryotherapy for Barrett's esophagus with high-grade dysplasia. Gastrointest Endosc. 2010;71:680–5.

62. Bisschops R. Optimal endoluminal treatment of Barrett's esophagus: integrating novel strategies into clinical practice. Expert Rev Gastroenterol Hepatol. 2011;4:319–33.
63. Hubbard N, Velanovich V. Endoscopic endoluminal radiofrequency ablation of Barrett's esophagus in patients with fundoplications. Surg Endosc. 2007;21:625–8.
64. Goers TA, Leao P, Cassera MA, et al. Ablation and laparoscopic reflux operative results in more effective and efficient treatment of Barrett's esophagus. J Am Coll Surg. 2011;213:486–92.
65. O'Connell K, Velanovich V. Effects of Nissen fundoplication on endoscopic endoluminal radiofrequency ablation of Barrett's esophagus. Surg Endosc. 2011;25:830–4.
66. Krishnan K, Pandolfino JE, Kahrilas PJ, et al. Increased risk for persistent intestinal metaplasia in patients with Barrett's esophagus and uncontrolled reflux exposure before radiofrequency ablation. Gastroenterology. 2012;143:576–81.
67. Rice TW, Sontag SJ. Debate: esophagectomy is the treatment of choice for high grade dysplasia in Barrett's esophagus. Am J Gastroenterol. 2006;101:2177–84.
68. Williams VA, Watson TJ, Herbella FA, et al. Esophagectomy for high-grade dysplasia is safe, curative and results in good alimentary outcome. J Gastrointest Surg. 2007;11:1589–97.
69. Djarv T, Lagegren J, Blazeby JM, Lagegren P. Long-term health-related quality of life following surgery for oesophageal cancer. Br J Surg. 2008;95:1121–6.
70. DeMeester SR. Vagal-sparing esophagectomy: is it a useful addition? Ann Thorac Surg. 2010;89:S2156–8.
71. Tsiouris A, Hammoud Z, Velanovich V. Barrett's esophagus after resection of the gastroesophageal junction: effects of concomitant fundoplication. World J Surg. 2011;35:1867–72.

Approach to Esophageal Strictures and Diverticula

12

Ciro Andolfi and P. Marco Fisichella

Esophageal Strictures

Introduction

Esophageal strictures are a quite common problem and are largely divided into benign and malignant types. Recent data shows that the overall incidence of new and recurrent esophageal strictures have decreased by 10% and 30%, respectively, over the last decade [1]. This incidence drop is most likely due to a decline in peptic-related strictures from the use of acid reducing medications, such as proton pump inhibitors (PPIs) [2]. However, it appears to be an increase in malignant strictures related to esophageal cancer, especially at the gastroesophageal junction [1]. Esophageal strictures can also be grouped into the three following categories: (1) intrinsic diseases (inflammation, fibrosis, or neoplasia); (2) extrinsic diseases (direct invasion or lymph node enlargement); and (3) diseases that disrupt esophageal peristalsis and/or lower esophageal sphincter (LES) function. The etiology of esophageal stricture can usually be identified using radiologic modalities and can be confirmed by endoscopic visualization and tissue biopsy. Use of manometry is critical when motility disorders are suspected [3]. Computed tomography (CT) and endoscopic ultrasound are valuable aids in staging of malignant strictures.

C. Andolfi, M.D.
Department of Surgery, The University of Chicago Pritzker School of Medicine, Chicago, IL, USA

P. M. Fisichella, M.D., M.B.A., F.A.C.S. (✉)
Department of Surgery, Brigham and Women's Hospital and Boston VA Healthcare System, Harvard Medical School, Boston, MA, USA
e-mail: piero.fisichella@va.gov

© Springer International Publishing AG, part of Springer Nature 2018
D. Oleynikov, P. M. Fisichella (eds.), *A Mastery Approach to Complex Esophageal Diseases*, https://doi.org/10.1007/978-3-319-75795-7_12

Etiology, Clinical Presentation and Diagnostic Procedures

Most benign esophageal strictures are caused by chronic inflammation leading to ulceration, formation of fibrous tissue, and collagen deposition. In the US, gastro-esophageal reflux disease (GERD) is the most common cause of benign esophageal strictures [1, 4]. These strictures are typically located at the gastroesophageal junction and are relatively short in length. Other common causes of benign esophageal strictures include anastomotic strictures, radiation injury, caustic ingestions, Schatzki rings, and esophageal webs. Approximately 20–30% of esophageal strictures are due to malignancy [5]. Squamous cell carcinoma is related to heavy smoking and can arise from any part of the esophagus. In contrast, the typical adenocarcinoma is related to GERD and Barrett's esophagus, and is more commonly located towards the distal esophagus. Table 12.1 summarizes benign and malignant causes of esophageal strictures.

Dysphagia to solids, liquids, or both is the main presenting complaint of patients with esophageal strictures. Patients with peptic strictures may also present with heartburn, odynophagia, food impaction, weight loss, and chest pain. Atypical presentations include chronic cough and asthma secondary to aspiration of food or acid. When approaching a patient with dysphagia, a detailed history usually provides valuable insight as to the underlying cause of stricture. The two main tools that accurately identify the presence or absence of a stricture are barium esophagram and endoscopy. A barium esophagram provides an objective evidence of the esophageal anatomy before any intervention. This study also provides information about location, length, and diameter of the stricture and possible irregularities of the esophageal wall. The information obtained can complement endoscopic findings. Lesions, such as diverticula and paraesophageal hernias, that potentially may lead to increased risk of complications during endoscopy can be identified. In addition, this study may be more sensitive than endoscopy for detection of subtle narrowing of the esophagus. However, endoscopy remains the preferred technique needed in evaluating dysphagia. Flexible endoscopy provides a platform to visually inspect the entire esophagus and upper GI tract, accurately identify the location and appearance of a stricture, perform tissue sampling, and immediately treat a stricture using

Table 12.1 Causes of esophageal strictures

Benign strictures	Malignant strictures
Peptic stricture	Squamous cell carcinoma
Schatzki ring	Adenocarcinoma
Webs	Extrinsic compression (e.g. malignant mediastinal lymph node, lung cancer)
Postsurgical anastomosis	
Caustic injury	
Radiation injury	
Eosinophilic esophagitis	
Extrinsic compression (e.g. vascular compression)	

endoscopic dilation. CT scans can be used to stage malignancies that produce esophageal strictures. Endoscopic ultrasound (EUS) is the most accurate means of identifying the extent of local invasion of an esophageal malignancy. Twenty-four-hour esophageal pH monitoring may be helpful in evaluating and documenting the amount of reflux in patients who remain symptomatic despite treatment with PPIs or fundoplication. Esophageal manometry is used to evaluate any patient suspected of having esophageal dysmotility. It has to be used as a preoperative tool before antireflux surgery to evaluate the presence of severe esophageal dysmotility.

Management

Traditionally, when managing peptic strictures more emphasis has been placed on mechanical dilatation, and coexistent esophagitis has been relatively ignored. However, several studies have demonstrated that aggressive acid suppression using PPIs is extremely beneficial in the initial treatment of esophageal stricture, as well as long-term management. A dysphagia score developed by Dakkak et al. in a study of 64 patients revealed that the stricture diameter only contributed to 30% of the dysphagia score and that esophagitis and other factors accounted for 70% of the score [6]. Smith et al. showed in a randomized study of 366 patients that omeprazole 20 mg/day was superior to ranitidine 300 mg twice a day in preventing stricture recurrence with re-dilation rates of 30% and 46%, respectively, at 12 months [7]. Accordingly, Marks et al. showed that the re-dilation rate in patients treated with omeprazole 20–40 mg/day was 41% versus 73% in patients treated with ranitidine 150–300 mg twice per day. Moreover, the omeprazole group showed higher rates of dysphagia relief and healing of esophagitis when compared with H_2 blockers [8].

The type of dilation technique is dependent on many factors, such as stricture characteristics, patient tolerance, and experience. No clear consensus exists; therefore, the type of procedure should be tailored individually. Three types of dilators are currently used. Mercury-filled bougies, such as Maloney or Hurst dilators, are designated for uncomplicated strictures with diameters greater than 12 mm. Dilation can be performed without fluoroscopic guidance, and minimal or no sedation is needed. Wire-guided polyvinyl bougies, such as Savary-Gilliard and American dilators, are rigid and suitable for longer and stiffer strictures. Fluoroscopy is performed most of the times. The range is 5–20 mm and dilators are reusable. Side effects include trauma to the larynx and pain. American dilators are shorter and impregnated with barium for better fluoroscopic visualization. Savary dilators are safe and effective and regularly used for pediatric eosinophilic esophagitis (EoE). In a retrospective study of 50 pediatric cases of EoE in which 11 cases had esophageal narrowing, dilation resulted in good response in all cases and the esophageal size improved from a 7 to 13.4 mm [9]. Through-the-scope (TTS) balloon dilators are used through the endoscope, and they allow for direct visualization. Fluoroscopy is not mandatory, but it is frequently performed. There is still a debate about the benefits of balloon dilators compared to Savary dilators. Two separate retrospective studies indicate that fluoroscopic balloon dilatation (FBD) is safe for treating esophageal anastomotic strictures after surgical repair and caustic esophageal strictures. Thyoka et al. reviewed 12-years data from 103 consecutive patients with esophageal anastomotic stricture following surgical repair who underwent 378 FBD sessions. Ninety-three patients (90%) achieved symptomatic relief. Of ten patients who underwent more procedures, three had stent placement, three had stricture resection, and four had esophageal reconstruction [10]. Uygun et al. reviewed 8 years' data from 38 children who underwent FBD for caustic esophageal stricture, 369 FBD sessions were successful overall. Patients who underwent FBD earlier following caustic ingestion had significantly faster and shorter treatment [11]. In a prospective, randomized study with 17 patients in each arm comparing balloon dilators with Savary dilators performed over a 2-year period, with the end point being 45F, stricture recurrence was similar in the first year but lower in the second year for balloons, fewer sessions were needed for balloons and less procedural discomfort occurred [12]. No consensus exists regarding the end point of esophageal dilation for peptic strictures. Most patients experience complete relief when dilated to 40–54F. Therefore, using this end point as a benchmark is recommended.

Limited data exist showing that intra-lesional steroid injection of peptic strictures may be beneficial. The mechanism is unclear; it may inhibit collagen formation and enhance collagen degradation, thus increasing stricture compliance. Triamcinolone 10 mg/mL in 0.5 mL was injected in four quadrants in two patients with a successful outcome as reported by Kirsch et al. [13]. Also, Lee et al. showed successful data achieving greater luminal diameters and duration between dilations in a nonrandomized cohort of patients with strictures of varying etiologies [14]. Similar results were obtained by Kochhar et al. in 71 patients with the injections of 20 mg of triamcinolone [15]. A randomized prospective trial of Savary dilation with or without intralesional steroids was conducted in 42 patients by Dunne et al.; it demonstrated a decreased need for second dilations in the steroid group at 1 year [16]. Similar results were seen in a study by Ramage et al. in 30 patients. Therefore, a trial of steroid injection may be reasonable in patients with benign strictures who experience no significant relief of dysphagia despite repeated dilations and aggressive antireflux therapy [17]. Hishiki et al. reported the use of repeated endoscopic dilatation with systemic steroids in a child with severe esophageal anastomotic stricture that did not respond to endoscopic dilatation and local steroid injection of the stricture. At 18 months' follow-up, the child remained asymptomatic without any further endoscopic dilations [18].

Repici et al presented a case series of 15 patients whose condition had failed endoscopic therapy. A temporary placement of an expandable polyester silicone-covered stent for 6 weeks was successful in 12 patients over a long-term period [19]. Still, the duration of stent placement is unclear, as strictures can recur after stent removal. More recently, biodegradable stents have shown some promise in animal studies [20].

There are limited options for patients with strictures who do not respond to endoscopic treatment. Surgery may be considered on a case-by-case basis. Unfortunately, the underlying etiology (e.g. radiation or caustic injury) makes surgical reconstruction technically challenging. Indications for surgery in peptic stricture include failed aggressive medical therapy or an unsuitable candidate for conservative treatment. This is usually a rare occurrence in the era of PPIs therapy.

Various procedures advocated include the following:

- Esophageal-sparing procedures: Standard antireflux surgery (total or partial) and esophageal lengthening with antireflux surgery (Collis-Nissen or Belsey gastroplasty).
- Esophageal resection and reconstruction with gastric or colon interposition.

If the benign peptic stricture is dilatable, an esophageal-sparing operation is preferred.

Esophageal Diverticula

Introduction

Esophageal diverticula are outpouchings of the esophagus that are classified according to site, etiology, and layers of the esophagus involved. According to the site they are termed pharyngoesophageal, parabronchial, or epiphrenic. They can be termed true when the entire thickness of the esophageal wall is involved or false when only the mucosa/submucosa is involved. Finally, they can be caused by pulsion related to increased intraluminal pressure or traction applied by structures external to the esophagus. Traction diverticula were usually caused by mediastinal lymph node involvement in tuberculosis with resultant fibrosis. Nowadays, traction diverticula are rare because of tuberculosis treatment. Pulsion diverticula are often caused by underlying motility disorders, and they can be identified by a barium swallow.

Clinical Presentation and Diagnostic Procedures

Many patients relate a history of dysphagia, chest pain, or regurgitation. Although physical examination findings are often normal and the diagnosis is made incidentally through radiographic studies and upper endoscopy, Zenker diverticula may present as a neck mass. Halitosis is due to accumulated food debris within the diverticulum. On standard chest radiographs and CT scans, large diverticula of the esophagus and hypopharynx may also manifest as air-filled or fluid-filled structures communicating with the esophagus. Barium swallow generally is the diagnostic procedure of choice. In addition to being excellent at defining the structural appearance of diverticula, barium swallow may also provide clues to underlying motility disturbances that may be involved in diverticular formation. Killian-Jamieson diverticula are sometimes detected on ultrasonography of the thyroid gland. Due to the proximity of the upper esophagus to the thyroid gland, pharyngoesophageal diverticula can mimic thyroid nodules on ultrasonography. Zenker diverticula reportedly can be distinguished from a thyroid nodule on ultrasound by the presence of air [21–23]. Esophageal manometry is critical to evaluate esophageal motility in these patients, especially if surgery is being considered [24]. It can also demonstrate the incoordination between the buccal squirt and relaxation of the cricopharyngeal muscle. High-resolution manometry (HRM) is a variant of the conventional manometry in which multiple recording sites are used, thus creating a map of the esophageal contractions. Esophagogastroduodenoscopy is essential to rule out mechanical conditions, such as strictures or neoplasms. Endoscopy is unnecessary in patients with Zenker diverticula if the diagnosis has been made using barium swallow. If an endoscopy is needed in a patient with Zenker, it should be performed with extreme caution to minimize the risk of perforation.

Management

Zenker's, or pharyngoesophageal, diverticula are the most common type. They are false, pulsion diverticula and occur in people older than 60 years as their pharyngeal muscle tone and elasticity decreases. They form in Killian's triangle between the pharyngeal constrictors and the cricopharyngeus muscle on the posterior side of the pharyngoesophageal junction. This is occasionally labeled as cricopharyngeal achalasia, since the cricopharyngeal muscle fails to relax. These patients may present with cough, increased salivation, dysphagia for solid foods, regurgitation, halitosis, chest pain, and respiratory distress. Sometimes, patients need to apply pressure to the neck to facilitate swallowing. Symptoms progress as the diverticulum enlarges and can lead to aspiration pneumonia [25]. The treatment for Zenker's diverticula is surgery. Many techniques are described; however, all involve a 7–10 cm extramucosal esophagomyotomy to ensure all cricopharyngeal fibers are transected. If the diverticulum is resected without esophagomyotomy, a fistula is likely to form. Because these diverticula are in the upper esophagus, a left cervical incision is used. Few surgeons opt for a transverse cervical incision. Typically, the diverticulum is completely resected; however, small residues may be left in place. Alternatively, it can be suspended to the surrounding tissue (diverticulopexy) to facilitate draining of contents. If GERD is present, a fundoplication should be taken into account.

Parabronchial, or midesophageal, diverticula were historically traction diverticula but are now more often due to pulsion or motility disorders. They are relatively wide and less than 5 cm in size. They are typically asymptomatic but can cause symptoms similar to those of Zenker's diverticula. Asymptomatic and minimally symptomatic esophageal body diverticula do not usually require treatment. In many patients with mid esophageal diverticula, dysphagia is related to the underlying dysmotility; thus, treatment should be directed to the dysmotility.

Epiphrenic, or supradiaphragmatic, diverticula occur within 10 cm of the gastroesophageal junction and are due to pulsion. They also are asymptomatic but can produce symptoms similar to the previous types. A distinguishing feature is the presence of epigastric pain. These also require investigation for motility disorders. They can be associated with trauma or congenital disorders such as Ehlers-Danlos. Surgical management of the patient with epiphrenic diverticulum includes three elements: myotomy, partial fundoplication, and possible diverticulectomy [26]. The goal of surgery is to address the underlying motility disorder, remove the diverticulum when appropriate, and prevent postoperative gastroesophageal reflux. Historically, a transthoracic approach through a left thoracotomy incision has been the standard of care. This allows optimal visualization and access to the distal esophagus and provides the best exposure for diverticulum resection, oversewing of the esophageal musculature, and myotomy. In the last decade, however, laparoscopy has become a reasonable approach for surgical management in most cases and has been shown in numerous clinical studies to be effective in providing symptomatic relief [27]. Regardless of whether treatment is done through an open, thoracoscopic, or laparoscopic approach, morbidity and mortality may be considerable. The most serious complication is esophageal leak either from the staple line or from missed mucosal disruption during myotomy. Sepsis, pneumonia, empyema, and abscess have lethal potential and should be addressed quickly when identified. Failure to perform an esophageal myotomy may result in high-pressure distal to the resected diverticulum, which can cause a leak with disruption of the staple line. Given its strategic location, an ED can be approached both from the chest and from the abdomen. Laparoscopy allows an easy approach to the upper abdomen, accessible creation of the myotomy, and partial fundoplication, while it spares the need for one-lung ventilation. However, these advantages may be limited in cases of a large size diverticulum, long distance between the diverticulum and the hiatus (8–10 cm), and dense adhesion in the mediastinum. In these circumstances, VATS may be more suitable as either single or combined procedures with laparoscopy.

References

1. El-Serag HB. Temporal trends in new and recurrent esophageal strictures in Department of Veterans Affairs. Am J Gastroenterol. 2006;101(8):1727–33.
2. Guda NM, Vakil N. Proton pump inhibitors and the time trends for esophageal dilation. Am J Gastroenterol. 2004;99(5):797–800.
3. Andolfi C, et al. Importance of esophageal manometry and pH monitoring in the evaluation of patients with refractory gastroesophageal reflux disease: a multicenter study. J Laparoendosc Adv Surg Tech A. 2016;26(7):548–50.
4. Spechler SJ. AGA technical review on treatment of patients with dysphagia caused by benign disorders of the distal esophagus. Gastroenterology. 1999;117(1):233–54.
5. Lew RJ, Kochman ML. A review of endoscopic methods of esophageal dilation. J Clin Gastroenterol. 2002;35(2):117–26.
6. Dakkak M, et al. Oesophagitis is as important as oesophageal stricture diameter in determining dysphagia. Gut. 1993;34(2):152–5.
7. Smith PM, et al. A comparison of omeprazole and ranitidine in the prevention of recurrence of benign esophageal stricture. Restore Investigator Group. Gastroenterology. 1994;107(5):1312–8.
8. Marks RD, et al. Omeprazole versus H2-receptor antagonists in treating patients with peptic stricture and esophagitis. Gastroenterology. 1994;106(4):907–15.
9. Al-Hussaini A. Savary dilation is safe and effective treatment for esophageal narrowing related to pediatric eosinophilic esophagitis. J Pediatr Gastroenterol Nutr. 2016;63(5):474–80.
10. Thyoka M, et al. Fluoroscopic balloon dilation of esophageal atresia anastomotic strictures in children and young adults: single-center study of 103 consecutive patients from 1999 to 2011. Radiology. 2014;271(2):596–601.

11. Uygun I, et al. Fluoroscopic balloon dilatation for caustic esophageal stricture in children: an 8-year experience. J Pediatr Surg. 2013;48(11):2230–4.
12. Saeed ZA, et al. Prospective randomized comparison of polyvinyl bougies and through-the-scope balloons for dilation of peptic strictures of the esophagus. Gastrointest Endosc. 1995;41(3):189–95.
13. Kirsch M, et al. Intralesional steroid injections for peptic esophageal strictures. Gastrointest Endosc. 1991;37(2):180–2.
14. Lee M, et al. Preliminary experience with endoscopic intralesional steroid injection therapy for refractory upper gastrointestinal strictures. Gastrointest Endosc. 1995;41(6):598–601.
15. Kochhar R, Makharia GK. Usefulness of intralesional triamcinolone in treatment of benign esophageal strictures. Gastrointest Endosc. 2002;56(6):829–34.
16. Dunne DP, Rupp T, Rex DK, Lehman GA. Five year follow-up of prospective randomized trial of Savary dilation with or without intralesional steroids for benign gastroesophageal reflux strictures. Gastroenterology. 1999;116:A152.
17. Ramage JI Jr, et al. A prospective, randomized, double-blind, placebo-controlled trial of endoscopic steroid injection therapy for recalcitrant esophageal peptic strictures. Am J Gastroenterol. 2005;100(11):2419–25.
18. Hishiki T, et al. Successful treatment of severe refractory anastomotic stricture in an infant after esophageal atresia repair by endoscopic balloon dilation combined with systemic administration of dexamethasone. Pediatr Surg Int. 2009;25(6):531–3.
19. Repici A, et al. Temporary placement of an expandable polyester silicone-covered stent for treatment of refractory benign esophageal strictures. Gastrointest Endosc. 2004;60(4):513–9.
20. Vandenplas Y, et al. A biodegradable esophageal stent in the treatment of a corrosive esophageal stenosis in a child. J Pediatr Gastroenterol Nutr. 2009;49(2):254–7.
21. Kim HK, et al. Characteristics of Killian-Jamieson diverticula mimicking a thyroid nodule. Head Neck. 2012;34(4):599–603.
22. Pang JC, et al. Killian-Jamieson diverticulum mimicking a suspicious thyroid nodule: sonographic diagnosis. J Clin Ultrasound. 2009;37(9):528–30.
23. Lixin J, et al. Sonographic diagnosis features of Zenker diverticulum. Eur J Radiol. 2011;80(2):e13–9.
24. Herbella FA, et al. Importance of esophageal manometry and pH monitoring for the evaluation of otorhinolaryngologic (ENT) manifestations of GERD. A multicenter study. J Gastrointest Surg. 2016;20(10):1673–8.
25. Andolfi C, et al. Achalasia and respiratory symptoms: effect of laparoscopic Heller myotomy. J Laparoendosc Adv Surg Tech A. 2016;26(9):675–9.
26. Andolfi C, Fisichella PM. Laparoscopic Heller myotomy and Dor fundoplication for esophageal achalasia: technique and perioperative management. J Laparoendosc Adv Surg Tech A. 2016;26(11):916–20.
27. Andolfi C, Wiesel O, Fisichella PM. Surgical treatment of epiphrenic diverticulum: technique and controversies. J Laparoendosc Adv Surg Tech A. 2016;26(11):905–10.

Esophageal Cancer

13

P. R. Boshier, A. Wirsching, and Donald E. Low

Introduction

Epidemiology

Esophageal cancer is a major global health burden affecting 746,000 individuals and responsible for 459,300 deaths in 2015 [1, 2]. In recent years the incidence of esophageal adenocarcinoma has risen significantly and is now the predominant subtype in North America and Europe [3]. For this reason esophageal adenocarcinoma will be the primary focus of this chapter.

Etiology and Screening

The preponderance of esophageal adenocarcinoma in Western populations is frequently attributed to concurrent high rates of visceral obesity and gastrointestinal reflux disease (GERD), the latter being associated with the development of Barrett's metaplasia, an initial step on the pathway to dysplasia and invasive malignancy. Other predisposing factors associated with the development of this tumor include Caucasian race, smoking and male gender. Appreciation for the influence of genetic phenotype is also widely accepted [4]. Compared to other cancers, esophageal adenocarcinoma has a high burden of point-mutations, particularly tumor suppressor genes including; TP53, CDK2NA and ARID1A [4]. Amplification of genes encoding the receptor tyrosine kinase, such as the human epidermal growth factor receptor 2 (HER2), is also commonly observed in patients with esophageal adenocarcinoma [4].

P. R. Boshier • A. Wirsching • D. E. Low (✉)
Department of Thoracic Surgery and Thoracic Oncology, Virginia Mason Medical Center, Seattle, WA, USA
e-mail: Donald.Low@virginiamason.org

© Springer International Publishing AG, part of Springer Nature 2018
D. Oleynikov, P. M. Fisichella (eds.), *A Mastery Approach to Complex Esophageal Diseases*, https://doi.org/10.1007/978-3-319-75795-7_13

With the exception of several high prevalence regions in China, no routine screening programs for esophageal cancer currently exist. Guidelines published by the American Gastroenterological Association and other leading bodies however recommend screening for Barrett's esophagus in high risk patients groups, including men over 50 years of age with long standing GERD (typically >5 years) especially where additional risk factors are present such as nocturnal reflux, hiatal hernia, smoking and centripetal obesity [5].

Diagnosis and Management

Clinical Presentation

Symptoms of early esophageal cancer are often vague and non-specific. They may therefore be mistaken for a number of benign conditions affecting the upper gastrointestinal tract. Common presenting symptoms of esophageal malignancy include progressive difficulty in swallowing (dysphagia), pain on swallowing (ondynophagia), unintended weight loss and heartburn that is unresponsive to medical therapy. Most clinicians would recommend that patients presenting with new onset dysphagia to solids that persists for greater than 10 days after starting antacid therapy should undergo upper gastrointestinal endoscopy. The presence of hoarseness, cough or pneumonia secondary to aspiration may signify laryngeal nerve compression or invasion by either the primary tumor or involved lymph nodes. Whilst hematemesis and melena are uncommon presentations, patients with esophageal cancer may be found to have iron deficiency anemia, secondary to occult bleeding. In a minority of patients esophageal cancer may be detected incidentally during investigation for an unrelated medical presentation or at the time of routine surveillance for Barrett's.

Diagnosis and Staging

Unless contraindicated, initial investigation of patients with suspected esophageal cancer should include endoscopy of the upper gastrointestinal tract. The benefit of this approach is the ability to directly visualize and obtain multiple biopsies of any mucosal lesions that are identified. Use of high-resolution endoscopy and narrow band imaging may also be used to enhance the detection of subtle lesions. At the time of endoscopy careful description of any lesions and their characteristic features should be made, as these are critically important when planning treatment. In cases where endoscopic examination is not available a double contrast barium study of the upper gastrointestinal tract may be considered [6].

Assessment of biopsies obtained at the time of endoscopy should report the histological subtype and tumor grade. Assessment of additional histochemical and immunohistochemical markers, including; cytokeratins, p63 and HER2, may also be required in order to fully characterize the tumor.

National Comprehensive Cancer Network (NCCN) guidelines recommend a detailed clinical history, physical examination, complete blood count and chemistry profile is undertaken in all patients presenting with newly diagnosed esophageal cancer [6]. Imaging with computerized tomography (CT) of the thorax and abdomen with oral and intravenous contrast should be performed to determine the presence of metastatic disease. Endoscopic ultrasound permits further assessment of both the depth of tumor invasion and possible lymph node involvement; both visually and through the use of ultrasound guided fine needle aspiration of suspicious nodes. In patients with no evidence of metastatic disease on CT, who are candidates for curative therapy, further evaluation with positron emission tomography (PET) is recommended owing to its superiority in detecting occult metastatic disease [7]. PET-CT has been shown to improve patient selection for curative surgery through its effect on modifying the recommendation of the multidisciplinary team in 38% of cases either by refuting earlier CT findings suspicious of metastatic disease or by identifying previously undetected metastatic disease and new lesions [8]. In addition, changes in PET findings as manifested by a decrease in tumor glucose metabolism in patients receiving neoadjuvant chemotherapy has been utilized to assess treatment response, prognosis and recurrence rate [9].

Staging laparoscopy and peritoneal cytology in patients with locally advanced adenocarcinoma at the gastroesophageal junction may also identify patients with occult peritoneal disease [10]. In our experience staging laparoscopy also offers an opportune moment for placement of a feeding jejunostomy tube or portacath, should this be indicated. Patients with tumors at or above the level of the carina in direct contact with the trachea or left main bronchus should be considered for bronchoscopy with biopsy or cytology of any abnormalities [6].

Additional investigations to be considered in patients, with specific indications, include: lung function tests; echocardiography, and; in cases where colonic interposition is being considered, endoscopic and angiographic assessment of the large bowel.

Staging Classification

The American Joint Committee on Cancer (AJCC) and the International Union for Cancer Control (UICC) TNM classification is used to categorize tumors, supporting treatment planning and prognostication [11]. Concerning gastroesophageal junction tumors, the new eighth edition of the TNM classification recognizes all tumors extending up to 2 cm into the gastric cardia as esophageal cancers and those tumors with an epicenter below this point as gastric cancers [11]. Whilst histological grade has not been included as part of the clinical or pathological TNM stage groups it is mandatory to report poorly differentiated- or signet cell tumor characteristics if present in a biopsy specimen as it can figure in treatment planning for early stage cancers.

Management of Esophageal Cancer

It should be emphasized that decisions regarding the management of esophageal cancer are best made within the setting of a multidisciplinary tumor board (MTB) with consideration given not only to disease stage but also patient's overall health and personal wishes. The recommendations of a MTB have been shown to differ from the managing providers initial plan in as many as one in four patients, emphasizing its important role within the care pathway of patients with esophageal cancer [12]. Discussion within the setting of a MTB has also been reported to increase the percentage of patients receiving complete staging and multidisciplinary evaluation whilst at the same time ensuring better adherence to nationally agreed care guidelines and significantly decreasing the interval between diagnosis and treatment [13].

Endoscopic Therapy

Small tumors that are limited to the mucosal epithelium (T1a, <2 cm) as well as Barrett's with high grade dysplasia should be considered for endoscopic mucosal resection (EMR) as first line therapy (Fig. 13.1). Limitations of this treatment approach in patients with early disease reflects the increasing risk of lymph node metastasis that is associated with depth of tumor invasion. In one large series overall 5-year survival rates were 91.5% in patients with intramucosal (T1a) adenocarcinoma [14]. It is important that patients receiving endoscopic treatment for high grade dysplasia or T1a adenocarcinoma undergo ablation of all remaining Barrett's epithelium so as to decrease the potential for metachronous cancers that can occur in approximately 15% of patients [14]. Total ablation of short segment Barrett's can be accomplished with EMR although stricture formation can occur if performed for circumferential lesions. Long segment Barrett's should be ablated with radiofrequency ablation [5].

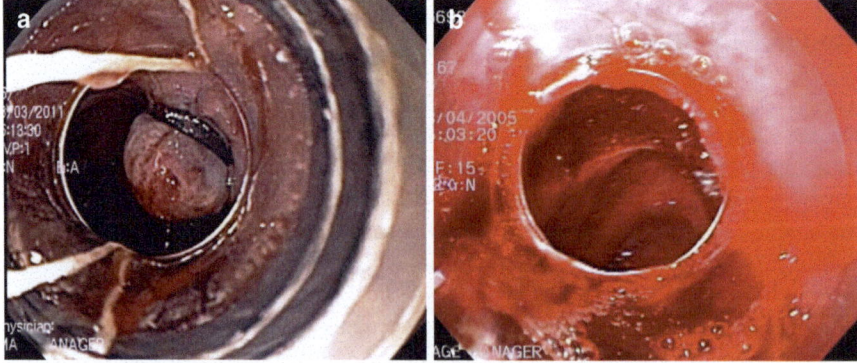

Fig. 13.1 Example of endoscopic mucosal resection of early esophageal cancer. Images demonstrate the site of the lesion (**a**) before and (**b**) after resection

There remains debate as to the suitability of patients with clinically staged T1b disease for endoscopic therapies. Whilst reported rates of lymph node metastasis in patients with T1a adenocarcinoma vary between 0% and 7%, up to 30% of patients with T1b disease may have nodal involvement [15–17]. Evidence suggests that in low risk T1b disease, characterized by submucosal invasion ≤500 µm, no lymphovascular invasion and well differentiated tumors, there may be a role for endoscopic mucosal resection with reported 5-year survival rates as high as 84% [18, 19]. Without evidence from randomized controlled trials comparing endoscopic therapies to surgery, the use of endoscopic therapy for disease that has extended into the submucosa shall remain controversial.

Chemotherapy and Chemoradiotherapy

The benefit of multimodal therapy in patients with esophageal cancer has been demonstrated in a number of randomized controlled trials. The Medical Research Council OEO2 trial is often regarded as the most influential study concerning the use of neoadjuvant chemotherapy in patients with esophageal cancer. In this study neoadjuvant chemotherapy (cisplatin and flurouracil) was associated with a significant survival advantage [20]. The subsequent MAGIC trial, that also included patients with gastric cancer, compared three cycles of epirubicin, cisplatin, and flurouracil both, before and after surgery versus surgery alone and similarly showed improved survival in those patients receiving chemotherapy [21].

Whilst neoadjuvant chemotherapy has historically been adopted within the United Kingdom, chemoradiotherapy is more widely used in the USA and other parts of the world. The most recent data from the Dutch CROSS trial reported superior 5-year survival in patients with esophageal and esophagogastric junctional tumors who received preoperative neoadjuvant chemoradiotherapy (carboplatin, paclitaxel and 41.4 Gy in 23 fractions) plus surgery versus surgery alone [22]. This survival benefit was strongly associated with squamous cell carcinoma but noted to a lesser degree in patients with adenocarcinoma [22]. The ongoing Neo-AEGIS and NExT trials are expected to provide further clarification of the value of neoadjuvant chemoradiotherapy in patients undergoing curative surgery for adenocarcinoma and squamous cell carcinoma, respectively.

A meta-analysis, comparing the outcomes of randomized controlled trials that investigated neoadjuvant chemotherapy or chemoradiotherapy versus surgery alone reported a significant survival benefit for both modalities of neoadjuvant therapy without being able to establish a clear advantage for either one over the other [23]. Concerns regarding the non-standardized oncological quality of surgery performed within randomized controlled trials for the treatment of gastroesophageal cancer have brought in to question the reliability of their findings [24].

Low and unpredictable rates of overall complete pathological response in patients receiving definitive chemotherapy without surgical resection, mean that at present there is no clear role for this therapy in the treatment of otherwise resectable esophageal cancer. Although definitive chemoradiotherapy has been shown to have a role in the management of esophageal squamous cell carcinoma, an equivalent finding is yet to be observed in patients with adenocarcinoma [25]. However, patients who undergo surgery following neoadjuvant chemoradiotherapy and demonstrate a complete pathological response have been found to have a significantly better long-term survival compared to patients with partial response [26]. A major challenge remains the ability to both predict and identify those patients who achieve complete response prior to definitive surgery. It is hoped that the ongoing preSANO trial, which aims to determine the accuracy of detecting the presence or absence of residual disease after neoadjuvant chemoradiotherapy, may yield further clarification of the role of this therapy in the setting of esophageal cancer [27].

Esophagectomy

Esophagectomy remains the primary curative therapy for patients with localized esophageal cancer. Surgical resection of the esophagus has traditionally been fraught with risks that are related both the unique technical challenges associated with this surgery as well as the physiological burden imposed upon often frail, elderly and malnourished patients. Major improvements in perioperative care during the last century have led to a consistent decline in early postoperative mortality following esophagectomy (Fig. 13.2) [28–34].

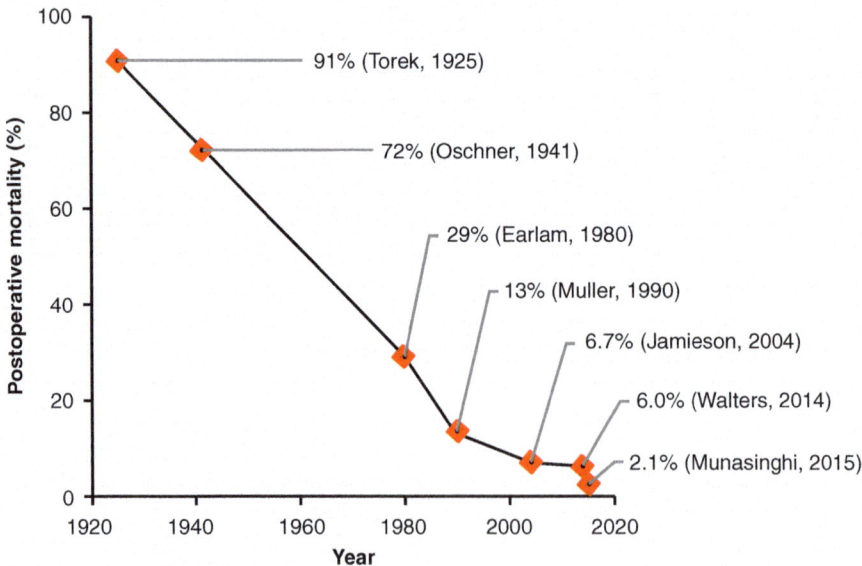

Fig. 13.2 Historical trend of early postoperative mortality after esophagectomy [28–33]

Surgical Principals of Esophagectomy

The intention of any operation for treatment of esophageal cancer should be to achieve curative R0 resection in a manner that best serves an individual's short- and long-term oncological and functional outcomes. Failure to achieve R0 resection is associated with inferior survival in patients with esophageal carcinoma [35].

A tendency for microscopic longitudinal spread of both adenocarcinomas and squamous cell carcinomas is promoted by the extensive lymphatic network within the esophageal submucosa. For adenocarcinomas of the esophagus a proximal resection margin of 10 cm and distal resection margin of 5 cm is advocated [36]. It is highly recommended that, where feasible, at least the proximal resection margin should be assessed with intraoperative frozen section. Involvement of the circumferential resection margin, defined as either; tumor at (College of American Pathologists) or within 1 mm (Royal College of Pathologists) of the margin has been associated with a worse prognosis following esophagectomy [37].

Extension of the dense submucosal lymphatic plexus to the surrounding tissues serve as a route for the early dissemination of esophageal cancers. In patients with tumors that have invaded into the submucosa (T1) there can be a 20% chance of spread to lymph nodes, rising to up to 60% in patients with tumors that invade the muscle of the esophageal wall (T2) [38]. As has been the case for many other solid-organ tumors, the extent of lymphadenectomy performed at the time of esophagectomy has been the subject of debate. Current opinion supports the practice of standardized lymphadenectomy as it has been shown to reduce the incidence of local recurrence and improves long-term survival [39–41]. Furthermore, extended lymphadenectomy also contributes to more accurate pathological staging. The extent of lymphadenectomy should be determined based on the location of the tumor within the esophagus as well as its histology [42]. Two field lymphadenectomy, is recommended for adenocarcinomas that commonly affect the lower third of the esophagus and metastasize to nodes within the lower mediastinum. This typically includes excision of both abdominal and thoracic lymph node stations (excluding stations 105 and 106) that are described in Table 13.1, as well as excision of the thoracic duct in selected cases. Extended two and three field lymphadenectomy, including lymph nodes in the upper mediastinum and cervical region, is often more appropriate for squamous cell carcinomas of the middle and upper third of the esophagus.

Higher lymph node yields are associated with greater overall survival [40, 43]. Whilst the optimum number of nodes that should be resected at the time of esophagectomy remains undetermined, there is evidence to suggest that for pT3/T4 tumors resection of ≥ 30 lymph nodes is optimal [43].

Surgical Approach to Esophageal Resection

The esophagus is a structure predominantly located within the posterior mediastinum where it lies in close proximity to many important structures, including the

Table 13.1 Esophageal lymph node stations

Cervical	Field Number	Laterality	Location
Lateral cervical	100	Left/right	Lateral
Cervical	101	Left/right	Paraesophageal
Supraclavicular	104	Left/right	Periesophageal
Thoracic			
Upper thoracic	105	Left/right	Paraesophageal
Pretracheal	106pre	–	Periesophageal
Tracheobronchial	106tb	Left/right	Periesophageal
Recurrent laryngeal nerve	106rec	Left/right	Periesophageal
Subcarinal	107	–	Periesophageal
Middle thoracic	108	Left/right	Paraesophageal
Main bronchus (hilar)	109	Left/right	Lateral
Lower thoracic	110	Left/right	Paraesophageal
Supradiaphragmatic	111	–	Paraesophageal
Posterior mediastinal	112	–	Paraesophageal
Abdominal			
Cardial	1	Right	Paraesophageal
Cardial	2	Left	Paraesophageal
Lesser curvature	3	–	Paraesophageal
Left gastric artery	7	–	Lateral
Common hepatic artery	8	–	Lateral
Celiac artery	9	–	Lateral
Splenic artery	11	–	Lateral
Diaphragmatic esophageal hiatus	20	–	Paraesophageal

heart, tracheobronchial tree, great vessels, thoracic duct, vagus and recurrent laryngeal nerves. Whilst the esophagus may be accessed in any number of ways including combinations of transthoracic, transhiatal and cervical approaches, no single method has been shown to be definitively superior.

Esophageal resection possess a unique challenge not only to the surgeon but also to the physiological reserve of patients. Resections that includes a transthoracic component to their approach typically affords the best access to the thoracic esophagus, however these operations have traditionally been associated with higher perioperative morbidity that is related to an extended operating time and the requirement for single lung ventilation [44].

Regardless of surgical approach, recent emphasis on standardization and centralization of care to high volume 'expert' centers has been shown to improve outcomes [33]. Assembly of multidisciplinary expertise and resources within centers where esophagectomy is regularly performed is believed to promote an environment wherein high quality outcomes become more predictable.

Open Esophagectomy

An open surgical procedure remains the most common method of performing esophagectomy. As previously discussed there are multiple potential approaches to the esophagus, which can involve access via one, two or three incisions. One characteristic that broadly separates these techniques from other gastrointestinal oncological procedures is the requirement for access through the wall of the thoracic cavity.

Transthoracic Esophagectomy

For tumors of the lower third of the esophagus and gastroesophageal junction the most widely used surgical approach is the two-phase (Ivor Lewis) procedure permitting subtotal esophagectomy. The initial phase of this procedure is accomplished via an upper midline incision with the patient in a supine position. During this stage the stomach is first mobilized and subsequently fashioned in to a tubular conduit after lymphadenectomy is completed (Fig. 13.3). As with all procedures that involve an abdominal stage there is the opportunity during this component of the operation

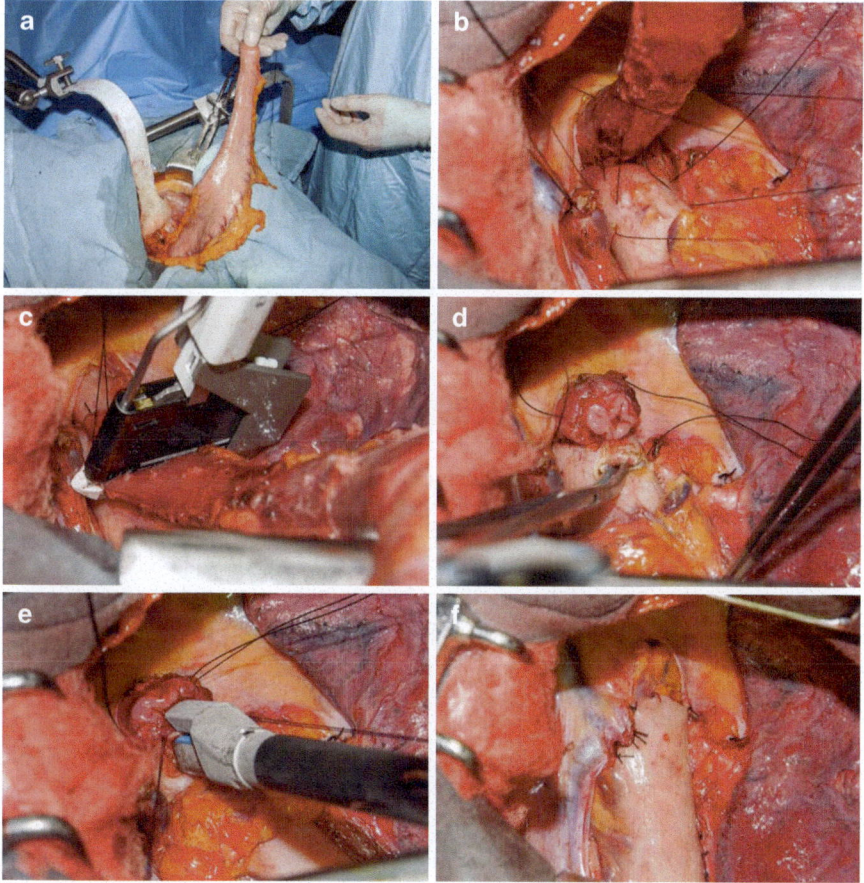

Fig. 13.3 Conduit formation and linearly stapled anastomotic technique performed during two-phase (Ivor Lewis) esophagectomy. (**a**) Gastric conduit formed during the abdominal stage; (**b**) apposition of native esophagus (superiorly) and gastric conduit (inferiorly); (**c**) transection of native esophagus; (**d**) formation of gastrotomy within conduit in preparation for (**e**) linear stapler device. (**f**) Resultant anastomosis overlaid with posterior mediastinal fat and the ligated azygos vein

for insertion of an intestinal feeding tube. After abdominal closure the patient is placed in a left lateral decubitus position and a right-sided posterolateral thoracotomy is performed in the fourth or fifth intercostal space. The right lung is collapsed to allow access to thoracic esophagus within the posterior mediastinum. Following completion of the resection and lymphadenectomy the gastric conduit is anastomosed to the proximal esophagus within the upper portion of the thoracic cavity, typically at or above the level of the azygos vein (Fig. 13.3). For tumors where an adequate proximal resection margin cannot be achieved via a two-phase approach, access to the cervical esophagus can be achieved via an additional neck incision. During this three phase (McKeown) approach the thoracic esophagus is mobilized via right posterolateral thoracotomy with subsequent abdominal and cervical phases permitting conduit formation and anastomosis within the neck. This approach also permits a directly visualized dissection of tumor adjacent to the trachea and three-field lymphadenectomy when indicated.

An alternative approach via a single left sided thoracoabdmoninal incision provides excellent exposure of the lower esophagus and upper abdomen. This approach can facilitate reconstruction with any type of conduit as the level of the anastomosis can be placed below or above the aortic arch or via a separate incision in the neck. This method of resection is considered best suited to tumors of the terminal esophagus and gastro-esophageal junction.

Transhiatal Esophagectomy

During transhiatal esophagectomy mobilization of the thoracic esophagus between abdominal and cervical incisions is achieved via a combination of both sharp dissection under vision and blind manual dissection. Following resection of the native esophagus a cervical anastomosis is performed. Whilst proponents of this procedure point to the high rates of morbidity that are associated with transthoracic approaches, many have concerns about the potential risks associated with the blind thoracic dissection as well as the adequacy of thoracic oncological resection. A lack of robust evidence from well-designed randomized controlled trials has meant that the superiority of either the trashiatal or transthoracic approach has not been conclusively demonstrated [44]. Complete 5-year survival data from one randomized controlled trial suggested no significant overall survival benefit for either approach [45]. For adenocarcinomas located within the distal esophagus there was a trend however towards superior survival in patients undergoing extended transthoracic esophagectomy.

Minimally Invasive Esophagectomy

During the last 25 years there has been a dramatic increase in the adoption of minimally invasive and hybrid techniques for esophageal resection. Current practice within international high volume centers submitting data to the Esophageal Complications Consensus Group indicated that minimally invasive esophagectomy is performed in almost 48% of esophageal resections (unpublished data).

Total minimally invasive esophagectomy by modified three-phase thoracoscopic, laparoscopic and open cervical approach has been extensively described by

Luketich [46]. The technical challenges of this procedure as well as concerns regarding higher rates of anastomotic leak and conduit necrosis have led others to seek alternative approaches. Many now favor two-phase and hybrid procedures that include either open thoracic (2-phase) or open abdominal (3-phase) techniques. The advantage of hybrid procedures is the ability for extracorporeal formation of the gastric conduit as well as a partial reduction in the learning curve. The potential benefits of thoracoscopic esophagectomy in the prone, as opposed to the traditional left lateral decubitus, position have also been reported in several cases series [47–49].

The results of the Dutch TIME trial suggested that minimally invasive esophagectomy is associated with lower rates of postoperative morbidity and improved quality of life [50]. Whilst lymph node harvest was comparable between open and minimally invasive techniques, the total number of lymph nodes retrieved in both groups was considered to be low [50]. Three-year follow-up from the TIME trial showed equivalent survival between both surgical groups [51]. At the time of writing the results of the French MIRO trial comparing a hybrid minimally invasive versus open esophagectomy have been made known, with findings indicating that there is a significant benefit of minimally invasive surgery in regard to intra- and postoperative morbidly and a non-significant trend towards better overall survival at 3-year [52, 53]. The most recent meta-analysis including the outcomes of 15,790 cases of resectable esophageal cancer demonstrated improved rates of early morbidity and mortality in patients undergoing minimally invasive procedures [54]. Ongoing clinical trials including one by the Japanese Clinical Oncology Group (JCOG1409) are expected to further determine the benefits of minimally invasive esophagectomy.

Surgeons have begun to explore the role of robotically assisted and fully robotic esophagectomy. Initial case series involving often small patient numbers have suggested that these approaches, at least in experienced centers, may yield equivalent early surgical and oncological outcomes compared to other minimally invasive techniques [55, 56].

Esophageal Reconstruction

Three factors that are important when approaching esophageal reconstruction at the time of esophagectomy are the type to conduit, the route of the conduit through the chest and the method of anastomosis. In the majority of esophagectomies performed worldwide a gastric conduit is considered most suitable for restoring continuity of the upper gastrointestinal tract due to its accessibility and the requirement for a single anastomosis. The conduit, formed from the greater curve of the stomach, should be free from the great omentum with fastidious attention to preserving the right gastroepiploic vascular arcade up until its termination. Ligation of the left gastroepiploic and short gastric vessels should then follow. Preservation of the right gastric vessels helps to maintain blood supply to the conduit via and intramural vascular network within the stomach. Determining the width of the conduit is often a matter of preference for individual surgeons. In our experience, fashioning a conduit approximately 3-4 cm in diameter provides both a reliable blood supply and helps prevent long-term functional disorders that may be linked to conduits of larger diameter (Fig. 13.3). At present there is no consensus evidence to support the use of a pyloric drainage procedure at the time of esophagectomy [57].

Alternative conduits can include either the large bowel or jejunum. A colonic conduit is most often used in circumstances where there is extensive tumor invasion of the stomach, a history of previous gastric resection or where a primary gastric conduit has failed.

There are three main routes by which the conduit can be passed to the proximal esophagus. The posterior mediastinal approach follows the natural course of the native esophagus and offers the shortest route from the abdomen to the upper thorax and neck. This route is obligated in all cases where the anastomosis is placed within the thoracic cavity. Alternative routes to the cervical esophagus are through either the anterior mediastinum (retrosternal) or subcutaenous tissue space (presternal). Whilst a presternal route is seldom used, the anterior mediastinum may offer a helpful alternative in cases where the posterior mediastinum has been compromised as a result of prior intervention or concurrent sepsis.

A large number of anastomotic techniques have been described and as in almost all other areas of esophageal surgery, operator preference is the defining feature of practice. Techniques can be broadly divided between hand sewn (one, two and three layer), circular stapled and linearly stapled (hybrid) procedures. Meta-analysis has suggested that anastomotic leak rate was less common when linearly stapled [58], but not circular stapled [59], techniques are used compared to hand sewn esophago-gastric anastomosis. In our experience a linearly stapled anastomosis is both technically straightforward and contributes to a reliable anastomosis and low rate of stricture formation (Fig. 13.3). Regardless of the method chosen, the fundamental principles governing the formation of any anastomosis dictate that there should be an adequate blood supply and a tension free anastomosis with attention paid to establishing an oncologically appropriate proximal and distal resection margin.

Perioperative Care and Management of Complications

The perioperative care of patients undergoing esophagectomy is the responsibility of the entire multidisciplinary team. An experienced multidisciplinary team will safeguard patients against adverse events and undertake physiological rescue when required. Efforts to protect patients from perioperative complications should begin at the time of their initial interaction with the esophagogastric care team. Patients should receive clear details of their expected treatment path and direct guidance as to nutritional and physical interventions that they can implement to build fortitude and cardiorespiratory reserve. The assessment and optimization of other comorbidities should also occur at this time. Consideration should be given to the potential benefits of preoperative supplementary nutrition, particularly in at risk patients who possess either low body mass index (<20 kg/m^2) or significant weight loss ($>5\%$ in 3-6 months).

Establishing adequate intraoperative monitoring and goal directed fluid therapy serves to avoid patients suffering physiological embarrassment. The central tenets of high quality perioperative anesthetic care are the preservation of organ perfusion, adherence to lung protective ventilation strategies and maintenance of adequate analgesia. Avoidance of excessive fluid administration aids in the recovery of gastrointestinal function and anastomotic healing as well as the prevention of respiratory complications. It is the responsibility of the surgical team to assist in this endeavor by preventing excessive blood loss at the time of surgery. Immediate extubation at the end of surgery should become the standard practice for all patients unless there is legitimate clinical concern regarding a patient's ability to maintain adequate spontaneous ventilation in the immediate postoperative period.

An understanding of the importance and benefits of standardized postoperative care has led many institutions to establish standardized care pathways for patients who are undergoing esophagectomy. Such pathways provide a roadmap for recovery allowing both clinicians and patients to predict and monitor progress. Evidence has shown that when implemented appropriately these pathways can have a positive influence on patient outcomes [60]. An outline of a postoperative clinical care pathway is

Table 13.2 Example of a postoperative care pathway

Postoperative day	Setting	Action/goal
0	ICU	• Sit up in bed • Maintain mean arterial blood pressure (MAP) <70 mmHg • Initiation of proton pump inhibitor therapy • Physical therapy visit, introduction to incentive spirometry
1	ICU/ ward	• Walks in corridor during the morning, subsequently walks 100–200 feet ×3 on day 1 • Stepdown from ICU care • Jejunal tube feeds started • Removal of apical chest drain in no air leak
2 onwards	Ward	• Walks 3–4 times per day, review by physical therapy • Titrate epidural to facilitate mobilization and maintenance of MAP >70 mmHg
3, 4 or 5	Ward	• Second chest drain removed (dependent on whether thoracic or cervical incision • Jejunal tube feeds increased to goal feeding
4 or 5	Ward	• Gastrograffin contrast swallow to assess gastric emptying and anastomotic integrity
5 or 6	Ward	• Removal of nasogastric tube • Removal of epidural • Conversation to enteral analgesia via oral or jejunal route • Jejunal tube feeds continued only at night • Commencement of oral liquid intake – limited to 1 cup per hour at discharge • Review by dietician with specific directions for advancement of oral nutrition over subsequent 3–4 weeks • Discharge planning with home help team
6 or 7	Ward	• Planned discharge

provided in Table 13.2. The Enhanced Recovery After Surgery (ERAS) society will shortly publish guidelines that are specific to esophageal surgery (unpublished data).

Despite advances in care, perioperative morbidity and mortality in patients undergoing surgery for esophageal cancer still remains amongst the highest of any oncological procedure. Inconsistency in the reporting of outcomes has meant that the true rate of complications is not known [8], but conservative estimates suggest that one in every two patients suffers morbidity [61, 62]. Recently published guidelines from the Esophagectomy Complications Consensus group (ECCG) now provide a basis for standardized data collection and reporting of outcomes [63]. Utilizing this standardized system for reporting, the ECCG, which includes 24 high volume esophagectomy centers, reported an overall complication rate of 59% (unpublished data). Greater appreciation of long-term functional disorder of the gastrointestinal tract are now also increasingly recognized [64].

Palliative Treatment in Advanced or Recurrent Esophageal Caner

A significant proportion of patients with esophageal cancer will present with advanced disease whilst many patients who undergo initial treatment with curative intent will suffer disease persistence or recurrence. It is therefore likely that the majority of patients with esophageal cancer will ultimately require palliation. In such circumstances local control of obstructive symptoms can often be achieved with stent placement or radiotherapy. Conventional partially covered metal stents can provide excellent palliation of dysphagia. Concurrent palliative chemotherapy offers the opportunity for systemic disease control and more effective (although modest) prolongation of survival.

Prognosis

Data from population based Surveillance, Epidemiology, and End Results cancer registries (SEER) in the United States suggest that the overall 5 year survival rate of patients with esophageal adenocarcinoma in the United States of America is approximately 19% [65]. For those patients with early or locally advanced disease overall survival following multimodal therapy was 47% at 5 years in the CROSS trial [22]. In the same study 5-year survival in patients undergoing only curative surgical resection was 33%. In patients with inoperable disease median survival seldom exceeds 1 year.

References

1. GBD 2015 Mortality and Causes of Death Collaborators. Global, regional, and national life expectancy, all-cause mortality, and cause-specific mortality for 249 causes of death, 1980–2015: a systematic analysis for the Global Burden of Disease Study 2015. Lancet. 2016;388(10053):1459–544.
2. GBD 2015 Disease and Injury Incidence and Prevalence Collaborators. Global, regional, and national incidence, prevalence, and years lived with disability for 310 diseases and injuries, 1990-2015: a systematic analysis for the Global Burden of Disease Study 2015. Lancet. 2016;388(10053):1545–602.
3. Hur C, Miller M, Kong CY, Dowling EC, Nattinger KJ, Dunn M, et al. Trends in esophageal adenocarcinoma incidence and mortality. Cancer. 2013;119(6):1149–58.
4. Smyth EC, Lagergren J, Fitzgerald RC, Lordick F, Shah MA, Lagergren P, et al. Oesophageal cancer. Nat Rev Dis Primers. 2017;3:17048.
5. Shaheen NJ, Falk GW, Iyer PG, Gerson LB. American College of G. ACG Clinical Guideline: diagnosis and management of Barrett's esophagus. Am J Gastroenterol. 2016;111(1):30–50; quiz 1.
6. NCCN. National Comprehensive Cancer Network Clinical Practice Guidelines in Oncology, Esophageal and Esophagogastric Junction Cancers Version 3. https://www.nccn.org/professionals/physician_gls/pdf/esophageal.pdf (2017). Accessed 21 Sep 2017.
7. Smyth E, Schoder H, Strong VE, Capanu M, Kelsen DP, Coit DG, et al. A prospective evaluation of the utility of 2-deoxy-2-[(18) F]fluoro-D-glucose positron emission tomography and computed tomography in staging locally advanced gastric cancer. Cancer. 2012;118(22):5481–8.
8. Blencowe NS, Whistance RN, Strong S, Hotton EJ, Ganesh S, Roach H, et al. Evaluating the role of fluorodeoxyglucose positron emission tomography-computed tomography in multi-disciplinary team recommendations for oesophago-gastric cancer. Br J Cancer. 2013;109(6):1445–50.
9. Ott K, Weber WA, Lordick F, Becker K, Busch R, Herrmann K, et al. Metabolic imaging predicts response, survival, and recurrence in adenocarcinomas of the esophagogastric junction. J Clin Oncol. 2006;24(29):4692–8.
10. Convie L, Thompson RJ, Kennedy R, Clements WD, Carey PD, Kennedy JA. The current role of staging laparoscopy in oesophagogastric cancer. Ann R Coll Surg Engl. 2015;97(2):146–50.
11. Rice T, Kelsen DP, Blackstone EH, et al. Esophagus and esophagogastric junction. In: Amin MB, Edge S, Greene FL, et al., editors. AJCC cancer staging manual. 8th ed. New York, NY: Springer Science+Business Media; 2016. p. 185–202.
12. Schmidt HM, Roberts JM, Bodnar AM, Kunz S, Kirtland SH, Koehler RP, et al. Thoracic multidisciplinary tumor board routinely impacts therapeutic plans in patients with lung and esophageal cancer: a prospective cohort study. Ann Thorac Surg. 2015;99(5):1719–24.
13. Freeman RK, Van Woerkom JM, Vyverberg A, Ascioti AJ. The effect of a multidisciplinary thoracic malignancy conference on the treatment of patients with esophageal cancer. Ann Thorac Surg. 2011;92(4):1239–42; discussion 43.
14. Pech O, May A, Manner H, Behrens A, Pohl J, Weferling M, et al. Long-term efficacy and safety of endoscopic resection for patients with mucosal adenocarcinoma of the esophagus. Gastroenterology. 2014;146(3):652–60. e1.
15. Leers JM, DeMeester SR, Oezcelik A, Klipfel N, Ayazi S, Abate E, et al. The prevalence of lymph node metastases in patients with T1 esophageal adenocarcinoma a retrospective review of esophagectomy specimens. Ann Surg. 2011;253(2):271–8.
16. Pennathur A, Farkas A, Krasinskas AM, Ferson PF, Gooding WE, Gibson MK, et al. Esophagectomy for T1 esophageal cancer: outcomes in 100 patients and implications for endoscopic therapy. Ann Thorac Surg. 2009;87(4):1048–54; discussion 54-5.
17. Sepesi B, Watson TJ, Zhou D, Polomsky M, Litle VR, Jones CE, et al. Are endoscopic therapies appropriate for superficial submucosal esophageal adenocarcinoma? An analysis of esophagectomy specimens. J Am Coll Surg. 2010;210(4):418–27.

18. Boys JA, Worrell SG, Chandrasoma P, Vallone JG, Maru DM, Zhang L, et al. Can the risk of lymph node metastases be gauged in endoscopically resected submucosal esophageal adeno-carcinomas? A multi-center study. J Gastrointest Surg. 2016;20(1):6–12; discussion.
19. Manner H, Pech O, Heldmann Y, May A, Pohl J, Behrens A, et al. Efficacy, safety, and long-term results of endoscopic treatment for early stage adenocarcinoma of the esophagus with low-risk sm1 invasion. Clin Gastroenterol Hepatol. 2013;11(6):630–5; quiz e45.
20. Medical Research Council Oesophageal Cancer Working Group. Surgical resection with or without preoperative chemotherapy in oesophageal cancer: a randomised controlled trial. Lancet. 2002;359(9319):1727–33.
21. Cunningham D, Allum WH, Stenning SP, Thompson JN, Van de Velde CJ, Nicolson M, et al. Perioperative chemotherapy versus surgery alone for resectable gastroesophageal cancer. N Engl J Med. 2006;355(1):11–20.
22. Shapiro J, van Lanschot JJB, Hulshof M, van Hagen P, van Berge Henegouwen MI, Wijnhoven BPL, et al. Neoadjuvant chemoradiotherapy plus surgery versus surgery alone for oesopha-geal or junctional cancer (CROSS): long-term results of a randomised controlled trial. Lancet Oncol. 2015;16(9):1090–8.
23. Sjoquist KM, Burmeister BH, Smithers BM, Zalcberg JR, Simes RJ, Barbour A, et al. Survival after neoadjuvant chemotherapy or chemoradiotherapy for resectable oesophageal carcinoma: an updated meta-analysis. Lancet Oncol. 2011;12(7):681–92.
24. Markar SR, Wiggins T, Ni M, Steyerberg EW, Van Lanschot JJ, Sasako M, et al. Assessment of the quality of surgery within randomised controlled trials for the treatment of gastro-oesophageal cancer: a systematic review. Lancet Oncol. 2015;16(1):e23–31.
25. Best LM, Mughal M, Gurusamy KS. Non-surgical versus surgical treatment for oesophageal cancer. Cochrane Database Syst Rev. 2016;3:CD011498.
26. Donahue JM, Nichols FC, Li Z, Schomas DA, Allen MS, Cassivi SD, et al. Complete patho-logic response after neoadjuvant chemoradiotherapy for esophageal cancer is associated with enhanced survival. Ann Thorac Surg. 2009;87(2):392–8; discussion 8-9.
27. Noordman BJ, Shapiro J, Spaander MC, Krishnadath KK, van Laarhoven HW, van Berge Henegouwen MI, et al. Accuracy of detecting residual disease after cross neoadjuvant chemo-radiotherapy for esophageal cancer (preSANO trial): rationale and protocol. JMIR Res Protoc. 2015;4(2):e79.
28. Torek F. Carcinoma of the thoracic portion of the esophagus. Arch Surg. 1925;10:353–60.
29. Oschner A, DeBakey M. Surgical aspects of carcinoma of the esophagus. J Thorac Surg. 1941;10:401–45.
30. Earlam R, Cunha-Melo JR. Oesophageal squamous cell carcinoma: I. A critical review of surgery. Br J Surg. 1980;67(6):381–90.
31. Muller JM, Erasmi H, Stelzner M, Zieren U, Pichlmaier H. Surgical therapy of oesophageal carcinoma. Br J Surg. 1990;77(8):845–57.
32. Jamieson GG, Mathew G, Ludemann R, Wayman J, Myers JC, Devitt PG. Postoperative mortal-ity following oesophagectomy and problems in reporting its rate. Br J Surg. 2004;91(8):943–7.
33. Munasinghe A, Markar SR, Mamidanna R, Darzi AW, Faiz OD, Hanna GB, et al. Is it time to centralize high-risk cancer care in the United States? Comparison of outcomes of esophagec-tomy between England and the United States. Ann Surg. 2015;262(1):79–85.
34. Walters DM, McMurry TL, Isbell JM, Stukenborg GJ, Kozower BD. Understanding mortality as a quality indicator after esophagectomy. Ann Thorac Surg. 2014;98(2):506–11; discussion 11-2.
35. Gertler R, Richter J, Stecher L, Nitsche U, Feith M. What to do after R1-resection of adeno-carcinomas of the esophagogastric junction? J Surg Oncol. 2016;114(4):428–33.
36. Migliore M, Rassl D, Criscione A. Longitudinal and circumferential resection margin in ade-nocarcinoma of distal esophagus and cardia. Future Oncol. 2014;10(5):891–901.
37. Chan DS, Reid TD, Howell I, Lewis WG. Systematic review and meta-analysis of the influ-ence of circumferential resection margin involvement on survival in patients with operable oesophageal cancer. Br J Surg. 2013;100(4):456–64.

38. Giugliano DN, Berger AC, Pucci MJ, Rosato EL, Evans NR, Meidl H, et al. Comparative quantitative lymph node assessment in localized esophageal cancer patients after R0 resection with and without neoadjuvant chemoradiation therapy. J Gastrointest Surg. 2017;21(9):1377–84.
39. Visser E, van Rossum PSN, Ruurda JP, van Hillegersberg R. Impact of lymph node yield on overall survival in patients treated with neoadjuvant chemoradiotherapy followed by esophagectomy for cancer: a population-based cohort study in the Netherlands. Ann Surg. 2017;266(5):863–9.
40. Peyre CG, Hagen JA, DeMeester SR, Altorki NK, Ancona E, Griffin SM, et al. The number of lymph nodes removed predicts survival in esophageal cancer: an international study on the impact of extent of surgical resection. Ann Surg. 2008;248(4):549–56.
41. Schwarz RE, Smith DD. Clinical impact of lymphadenectomy extent in resectable gastric cancer of advanced stage. Ann Surg Oncol. 2007;14(2):317–28.
42. Tachimori Y, Ozawa S, Numasaki H, Matsubara H, Shinoda M, Toh Y, et al. Efficacy of lymph node dissection by node zones according to tumor location for esophageal squamous cell carcinoma. Esophagus. 2016;13:1–7.
43. Rizk NP, Ishwaran H, Rice TW, Chen LQ, Schipper PH, Kesler KA, et al. Optimum lymphadenectomy for esophageal cancer. Ann Surg. 2010;251(1):46–50.
44. Boshier PR, Anderson O, Hanna GB. Transthoracic versus transhiatal esophagectomy for the treatment of esophagogastric cancer: a meta-analysis. Ann Surg. 2011;254(6):894–906.
45. Omloo JM, Lagarde SM, Hulscher JB, Reitsma JB, Fockens P, van Dekken H, et al. Extended transthoracic resection compared with limited transhiatal resection for adenocarcinoma of the mid/distal esophagus: five-year survival of a randomized clinical trial. Ann Surg. 2007;246(6):992–1000; discussion 1.
46. Luketich JD, Pennathur A, Awais O, Levy RM, Keeley S, Shende M, et al. Outcomes after minimally invasive esophagectomy: review of over 1000 patients. Ann Surg. 2012;256(1):95–103.
47. Fukuda N, Shichinohe T, Ebihara Y, Nakanishi Y, Asano T, Noji T, et al. Thoracoscopic esophagectomy in the prone position versus the lateral position (hand-assisted thoracoscopic surgery): a retrospective cohort study of 127 consecutive esophageal cancer patients. Surg Laparosc Endosc Percutan Tech. 2017;27(3):179–82.
48. Otsubo D, Nakamura T, Yamamoto M, Kanaji S, Kanemitsu K, Yamashita K, et al. Prone position in thoracoscopic esophagectomy improves postoperative oxygenation and reduces pulmonary complications. Surg Endosc. 2017;31(3):1136–41.
49. Teshima J, Miyata G, Kamei T, Nakano T, Abe S, Katsura K, et al. Comparison of short-term outcomes between prone and lateral decubitus positions for thoracoscopic esophagectomy. Surg Endosc. 2015;29(9):2756–62.
50. Biere SS, van Berge Henegouwen MI, Maas KW, Bonavina L, Rosman C, Garcia JR, et al. Minimally invasive versus open oesophagectomy for patients with oesophageal cancer: a multicentre, open-label, randomised controlled trial. Lancet. 2012;379(9829):1887–92.
51. Straatman J, van der Wielen N, Cuesta MA, Daams F, Roig Garcia J, Bonavina L, et al. Minimally invasive versus open esophageal resection: three-year follow-up of the previously reported randomized controlled trial: the TIME trial. Ann Surg. 2017;266(2):232–6.
52. Briez N, Piessen G, Bonnetain F, Brigand C, Carrere N, Collet D, et al. Open versus laparoscopically-assisted oesophagectomy for cancer: a multicentre randomised controlled phase III trial—the MIRO trial. BMC Cancer. 2011;11:310.
53. Mariette C, Markar SR, Dabakuyo-Yonli T, Meunier B, Pezet D, Collet D, et al. Abstract 615O; Hybrid minimally invasive vs. open esophagectomy for patients with esophageal cancer: long-term outcomes of a multicentre, open-label, randomized phase III controlled trial, the MIRO trial. ESMO 20172017.
54. Yibulayin W, Abulizi S, Lv H, Sun W. Minimally invasive oesophagectomy versus open esophagectomy for resectable esophageal cancer: a meta-analysis. World J Surg Oncol. 2016;14(1):304.
55. Okusanya OT, Sarkaria IS, Hess NR, Nason KS, Sanchez MV, Levy RM, et al. Robotic assisted minimally invasive esophagectomy (RAMIE): the University of Pittsburgh Medical Center initial experience. Ann Cardiothorac Surg. 2017;6(2):179–85.

56. Park S, Hwang Y, Lee HJ, Park IK, Kim YT, Kang CH. Comparison of robot-assisted esopha-
    gectomy and thoracoscopic esophagectomy in esophageal squamous cell carcinoma. J Thorac
    Dis. 2016;8(10):2853–61.
57. Arya S, Markar SR, Karthikesalingam A, Hanna GB. The impact of pyloric drainage on clinical
    outcome following esophagectomy: a systematic review. Dis Esophagus. 2015;28(4):326–35.
58. Deng XF, Liu QX, Zhou D, Min JX, Dai JG. Hand-sewn vs linearly stapled esophagogastric anas-
    tomosis for esophageal cancer: a meta-analysis. World J Gastroenterol. 2015;21(15):4757–64.
59. Wang Q, He XR, Shi CH, Tian JH, Jiang L, He SL, et al. Hand-Sewn versus stapled esopha-
    gogastric anastomosis in the neck: a systematic review and meta-analysis of randomized con-
    trolled trials. Indian J Surg. 2015;77(2):133–40.
60. Markar SR, Karthikesalingam A, Low DE. Enhanced recovery pathways lead to an improve-
    ment in postoperative outcomes following esophagectomy: systematic review and pooled
    analysis. Dis Esophagus. 2015;28(5):468–75.
61. Dunst CM, Swanstrom LL. Minimally invasive esophagectomy. J Gastrointest Surg.
    2010;14(Suppl 1):S108–14.
62. Merkow RP, Bilimoria KY, McCarter MD, Phillips JD, DeCamp MM, Sherman KL, et al.
    Short-term outcomes after esophagectomy at 164 American College of Surgeons National
    Surgical Quality Improvement Program hospitals: effect of operative approach and hospital-
    level variation. Arch Surg. 2012;147(11):1009–16.
63. Low DE, Alderson D, Cecconello I, Chang AC, Darling GE, D'Journo XB, et al.
    International consensus on standardization of data collection for complications associated
    with esophagectomy: Esophagectomy Complications Consensus Group (ECCG). Ann Surg.
    2015;262(2):286–94.
64. Irino T, Tsekrekos A, Coppola A, Scandavini CM, Shetye A, Lundell L, et al. Long-term func-
    tional outcomes after replacement of the esophagus with gastric, colonic, or jejunal conduits:
    a systematic literature review. Dis Esophagus. 2017;30(12):1–11.
65. NCI. National Cancer Institute; Surveillance, Epidemiology, and End Results Program. Cancer
    Stat Facts: Esophageal Cancer, https://seer.cancer.gov/statfacts/html/esoph.html. Accessed 21
    Sep 2017.

Index

© Springer International Publishing AG, part of Springer Nature 2018   183
D. Oleynikov, P. M. Fisichella (eds.), *A Mastery Approach to Complex*
Esophageal Diseases, https://doi.org/10.1007/978-3-319-75795-7

The manufacturer's authorised representative in the EU is Springer
Nature Customer Service Centre GmbH, Europaplatz 3, 69115 Heidelberg,
Germany. If you have any concerns regarding our products, please
contact ProductSafety@springernature.com

Printed and bound by CPI Group (UK) Ltd, Croydon, CR0 4YY

29/04/2026

02099516-0002